hashimoto's diet for the newly diagnosed

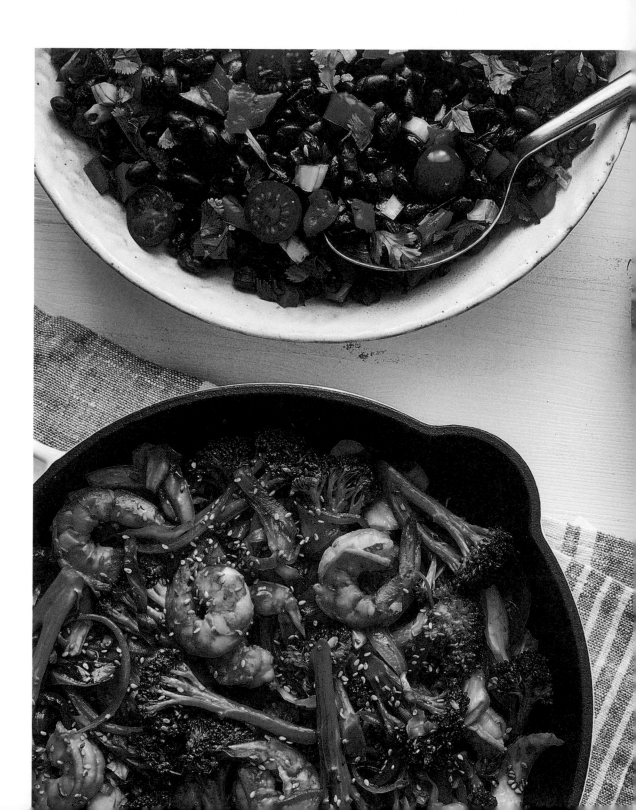

hashimoto's
diet for the
newly diagnosed

A 21-Day Elimination Diet Meal Plan and Cookbook

Daphne Olivier, LDN, RD, CDCES, IFNCP

photography by Hélène Dujardin

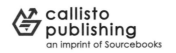
callisto
publishing
an imprint of Sourcebooks

Copyright © 2020 by Callisto Publishing LLC

Cover and internal design © 2020 by Callisto Publishing LLC

Photography © 2020 Hélène Dujardin. Food styling by Anna Hampton.

Author photo by Heather Renae Photography

Interior and Cover Designer: Carlos Esparza

Art Producer: Meg Baggott

Editor: Rachelle Cihonski

Production Editor: Emily Sheehan

Published by Callisto Publishing LLC C/O Sourcebooks LLC
P.O. Box 4410, Naperville, Illinois 60567-4410
(630) 961-3900
callistopublishing.com

Printed and Bound In China
OGP 13

This book is dedicated to those who have been struggling to feel better and more like themselves—and who recognize the power of food as a tool for improving the way they feel.

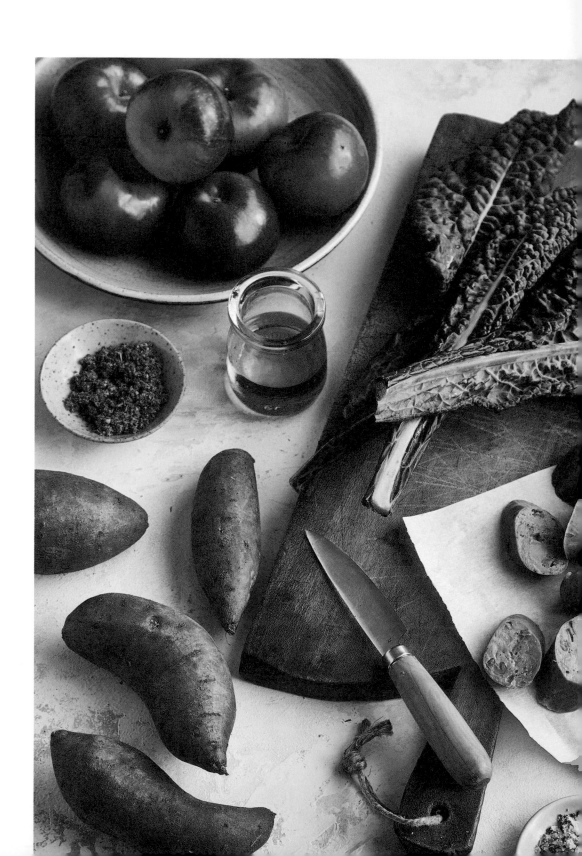

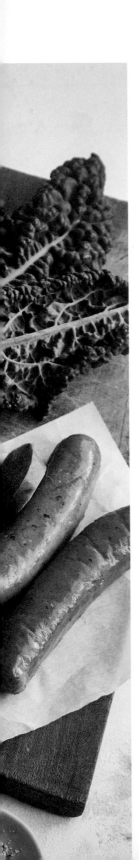

Contents

Introduction

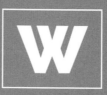

elcome! I am so happy you picked up this book in an effort to start moving toward being healthy. If you have been suffering from the symptoms of hormone imbalance fueled by Hashimoto's, and if you've been using only medications to manage your diagnosis so far, this book will help you understand your role in the disease and wellness process and how to make what you eat work in your favor. I know because I've been there.

From an early age, I always knew I wanted to be a dietitian. My family was the kind that talked about diets, ways to lower calories, foods that were calorie-free—all the things that come up when you have a dieting mentality. I thought this is what health was all about, and that I would be good at it because I knew what to do. Additionally, I started running when I was about eight years old, and always used that for both exercise and stress relief. Some version of health and wellness has always been a part of my life.

Despite the diets, though, members of my family have struggled with cancer, diabetes, heart disease, hypertension, obesity, hypothyroidism, and depression. I thought I was immune to all of that because of my healthy ways. Until 2014.

In January 2014 I had not been feeling like myself. I couldn't get enough sleep to make me feel rested, and I had a hard time getting excited about anything. I was gaining weight, had no sex drive, and generally felt like my head was in the clouds. Although I didn't have a "reason" to be depressed, I felt like what I'd always imagined depression was like—just going through the motions of life. I was ready to walk away from my nutrition practice that I'd worked so hard to build, and leave my very supportive husband and son to run away to a place where I had no responsibilities. I knew something was wrong, because this was *not* me.

One evening in May, my husband was out of town for work. After picking up my son from school, I dragged him to my office to finish up some work. Afterward, we agreed to go to a trendy pizza joint that had just opened. We each ate our personal pan pizza and the next day I felt like I had been hit by a truck. I was achy and tired, and my body felt heavy; I could not focus on anything, and my thinking was unproductive. I was unable to get much done that day, or for the following three days. I had a hunch as to what might be going on. During my upcoming annual doctor's visit, I asked to have a full thyroid panel run, including thyroid antibodies. My suspicion was right: a diagnosis of Hashimoto's thyroiditis. This was something I had been studying for many years, and a diagnosis I had worked through with many people in my practice, so I knew what I had to do.

Over the years I've researched, tweaked, and adjusted much of what I put into practice in my own life, which I've compiled in this book. My symptoms have resolved, although they do raise their head every now and then. Now that I know the cause of my familiar symptoms, I have the tools to quickly put them to rest.

This 21-day elimination diet is the first step, and the one you have most control over for putting yourself on the path to a healthy, symptom-free life. While this is not a substitute for working with your health practitioner, this book will outline how to begin the process of changing your eating habits and defining the diet that works uniquely for you. I've put it together in an easy format and provided you with all the tools you need to transition through an elimination diet, despite the fatigue, brain fog, and melancholy feelings you may be having. You *can* do this! Let's get started.

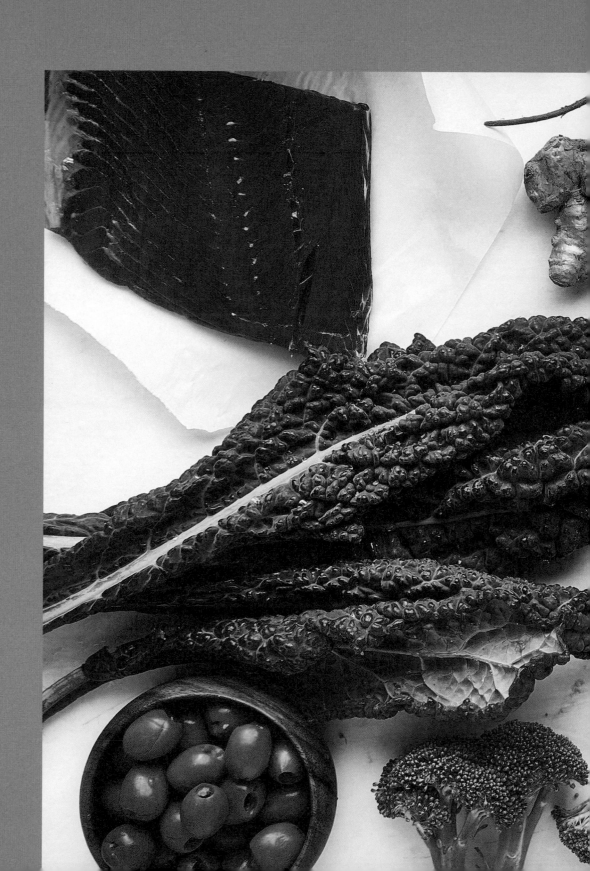

PART ONE

The Hashimoto's Diet Solution

Hashimoto's thyroiditis is a complex disease process that involves your gastrointestinal tract, your immune system, and your endocrine system. In this part you'll find an explanation of how it all works and why your diet plays a significant role in the process of healing. Then I'll help you get ready for the elimination diet with a step-by-step guide for how to prepare your kitchen—and your mindset.

The centerpiece of this part is the 21-day elimination diet meal plan, where you'll find everything from daily meals to weekly shopping lists. I'll explain how to systematically test which foods you can add back into your diet, and how to feel better about walking away from the foods that will not support your well-being.

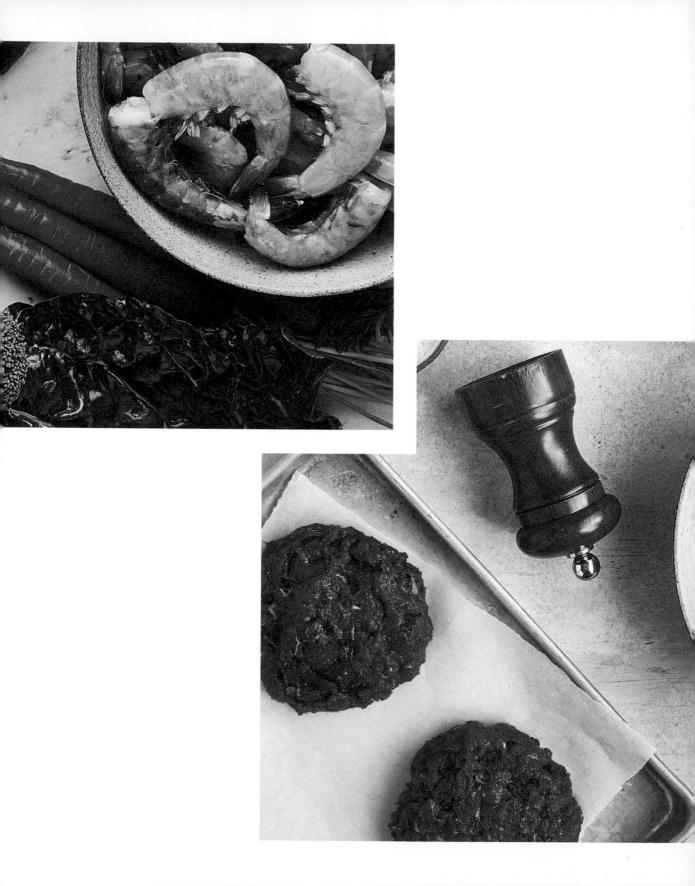

CHAPTER 1
Digesting Your Diagnosis

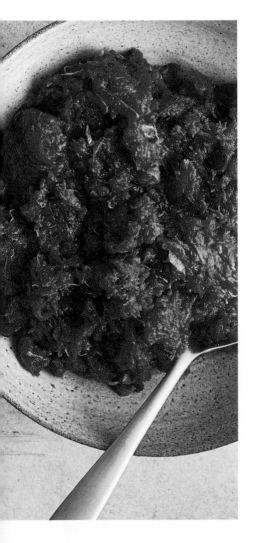

If you picked up this book, chances are you recently received a diagnosis that has changed your life and has potentially left you feeling confused, overwhelmed, or unsure of what to do next. Finally, your doctors have identified why you have been feeling so lousy. They've confirmed that what you've been feeling is real: The fatigue, brain fog, weight gain, constipation, hair falling out, feelings of melancholy—it's not all in your head. It's Hashimoto's thyroiditis. If you're wondering, "What now?" you've come to the right book.

A diagnosis is the first step on the road to healing. And while your medical team will serve as a great resource for you on this journey, it is *you* who plays the biggest role in your healing process. You have the power to make day-to-day changes that can increase your vitality and get you back to the "you" that you know is in there.

While there is relief in knowing there is a diagnosis to explain the way you feel, the steps to healing are not always easy. They require effort. They require patience. They require persistence. There is a lot to learn, but, without question, you can do it. I am here for you. My goal in this book is to break down this process into digestible steps so that you can move forward in your healing process and feel like yourself again. Let's get started.

Hashimoto's 101

Now that you have a Hashimoto's diagnosis, the next step is to understand what is going on in your body, specifically your immune system and your thyroid gland.

How the Immune System Works

The immune system is a complex system made up of organs, cells, and proteins, all of which play a crucial role in keeping you safe from the outside world. The immune system has three jobs:

1. Overcome pathogens—bacteria, viruses, and other microorganisms that cause disease—and remove them from the body
2. Neutralize toxins from the outside environment such as alcohol, chemicals from personal care products, and medications
3. Recognize and destroy the body's own renegade cells that would otherwise create illness, such as cancer cells

The immune system does this by recognizing proteins. The surfaces of bacteria, viruses, and other microorganisms have specific proteins called antigens. These proteins are made up of a detailed sequence of amino acids. You can think of them as a strand of pearls, each one with an identifiable shape. Once the immune system has been exposed to a microorganism, it will recognize the amino acid sequence, identify it as foreign material, and signal the body to destroy it.

Sometimes the immune system gets misguided and will mistake a part of itself for foreign material. This is called an autoimmune response. In some cases, the immune system will attack the whole body, such as in the case of systemic lupus erythematosus, but in other cases it will attack certain organs, such as the pancreas in type 1 diabetes, or the thyroid in Hashimoto's.

It is unclear what causes the immune system to misfire. Some theories suggest infections, while others suspect look-alike proteins found in foreign material and the self-body proteins. However, according to the work of Dr. Alessio Fasano, director of the Mucosal Immunology and Biology Research Center at Massachusetts General Hospital for Children, there are three things that are always present in autoimmune diseases: genetic predisposition; an environmental trigger such as a virus or protein; and intestinal permeability, also known as leaky gut.

The Role of the Thyroid

The thyroid is an endocrine gland that sits at the base of the neck. The pituitary gland, a tiny gland located in the brain's hypothalamus, sends a signal to the thyroid gland via thyroid stimulating hormone (TSH) to produce thyroid hormones. The principal hormone produced by the thyroid is T4, but your cells use a thyroid hormone called T3. This means your body must convert T4 into T3 for your cells to effectively use the hormone. These hormones are used by *every cell* in the body, and play a role in a plethora of metabolic functions, including regulating your metabolism and body weight, your heart rate, your body temperature, parts of your nervous system, your menstrual cycles, your blood sugar and insulin levels, and your cholesterol levels.

In addition, the thyroid gland works in conjunction with other endocrine glands and hormones, such as the adrenal gland and its hormones (including cortisol and adrenaline), the hormone insulin, and your reproductive hormones (estrogen, progesterone, and testosterone). As you can imagine, when the thyroid is not functioning at its best, it will affect the way the body functions in many ways.

When thyroid function is compromised through autoimmunity, it interferes with the gland's ability to produce hormones. The immune attack begins to destroy the thyroid gland and will slow down the production of thyroid hormone T4, which creates a cascading effect eventually leading to symptoms of hypothyroidism—low thyroid function. In fact, Hashimoto's is often treated as hypothyroidism, addressing the lack of hormones but missing the immune system involvement. Unless tested through labs that are specifically looking at antibodies against the thyroid, or an ultrasound, it can be misdiagnosed. If the immune attack against the thyroid does not stop, it will eventually destroy the thyroid gland completely, leaving it incapable of producing hormones on its own.

Causes and Symptoms of Hashimoto's

When thyroid hormone production is decreased, it causes symptoms of hypothyroidism. These symptoms are often subtle and can easily be blurred by general feelings of being overwhelmed, "the blues," and aging. Some of the most common symptoms of Hashimoto's, like symptoms of hypothyroidism, include weight gain, getting tired easily, sensitivity to cold, mental sluggishness or brain fog, daytime sleepiness, dry skin, and constipation.

It is unclear what exactly causes Hashimoto's; however, there are some theories. One theory is known as molecular mimicry. We talked about proteins being made up of amino acids in a sequence, like a strand of pearls with specific shapes. In molecular mimicry the amino acid sequence in the proteins of some foreign material, such as infectious bacteria, viruses, or gluten, looks very similar to the amino acid sequence of the thyroid gland. The immune system is triggered to attack the foreign material, and while it is activated it will accidentally mistake the thyroid for the foreign material and continue to attack. This creates a constant attack on the thyroid gland.

If the immune attack is not halted, later stages can increase the likelihood of developing other autoimmune diseases. This happens because the immune system is fired up and accidentally begins attacking other parts of the body. The most common autoimmune diseases linked to Hashimoto's disease include celiac disease, type 1 diabetes, and pernicious anemia, which affects the body's ability to make vitamin B12.

The Role of Diet

While the science can seem overwhelming, there is a silver lining: You play a big part in how your disease progresses. One way you can effectively manage your Hashimoto's is through diet. You have complete control over what you are eating every day.

Currently Hashimoto's has no cure; however, you *can* improve your thyroid function and prevent further thyroid disruption. One of the most potent tools in healing is food. After all, what you put into your body will affect the way the body functions. You want to use food in your favor, both by eliminating foods that could potentially cause an autoimmune response and by including foods that have the nutrients needed to effectively produce thyroid hormones.

By properly feeding your body, you can provide the nutrients needed to support your thyroid and influence your immune system. This will ensure that you are getting the specific nutrients that are vital to the production of thyroid hormones and support how each cell uses them. In addition, about 70 percent of your immune system lives in the gastrointestinal tract, which is where your food goes to be absorbed, so the right diet can support your immune system.

Using diet to influence your disease is done by adding some foods and eliminating others. While some foods are standard, everyone is very different. Through this step-by-step process you will fine-tune your diet to create your own personalized meal plan that takes into account how your body reacts.

The Link Between Food and Hashimoto's

Let's dive into how food affects your immune system. Think of your gastrointestinal tract as an open tube from top (mouth) to bottom (anus). This tube houses enzymes that break larger particles into smaller ones, such as the pearl strand of proteins into single amino acids. The tube also contains hormones, which act as messengers sending communication signals to organs and glands, and a complex system of immune modulators. These modulators are both inside the tube and immediately outside the tube, ready to detect what is beneficial and what is potentially harmful, and destroy anything deemed harmful.

In addition, this gastrointestinal tube is made up of one layer of cells that acts as the gatekeeper, determining what stays in the tube and what gets absorbed into the body. Naturally, the cells of this layer are held closely together, with the membrane of each cell touching one another. This connection is called a tight junction. When the cells are signaled, they separate, creating an opening that allows fatty acids, amino acids, glucose, vitamins, minerals, and phytochemicals to pass through the protective layer to be absorbed into the body.

When the tight junctions between cells are not held closely together it's known as intestinal permeability, or leaky gut. This is a problem because food particles that are not completely broken down, plus bacteria and viruses in the gut, have an easy passageway into the body. The immune system then gets involved to get rid of these foreign materials. All this activity "excites" the immune system, which goes on the attack, sometimes mistaking your own cells for foreign material.

The foods you eat can either build up the body or tear it down, so it is important to choose wisely. Some food proteins create a leaky gut. Some foods cause food sensitivities created by a complex inflammatory immune response. This low-grade inflammation can be thought of as a small fire that the immune system is constantly trying to extinguish. When you have continual low-grade inflammation, even without significant symptoms, harmless substances can become targets of the already excited immune system.

On the flip side, there are a variety of specific vitamins and minerals that are essential in calming the immune system and crucial in the production of thyroid hormones, increasing the body's ability to convert the T4 hormone to T3 and improving the way the cells use thyroid hormone. Choosing foods that will support these systems is critical in the healing process.

Common Triggers

There are a few common dietary triggers for many people with Hashimoto's. They can either trigger the immune system, or negatively affect the thyroid, the adrenal glands, estrogen balance, or blood sugar balance.

Gluten

Gluten is a protein found in grains and is known to cause intestinal permeability, commonly known as leaky gut. Remember when we talked about amino acids looking like a strand of pearls? When not completely digested, the gluten amino acid strand looks very similar to the thyroid amino acid strand. The body can get confused between gluten molecules and thyroid tissue, causing an attack on the thyroid.

Dairy

Dairy products have three components that may be challenging: lactose, casein, and whey. Lactose is a specific sugar that is broken down, or digested, by an enzyme called lactase. As we get older our body stops making this enzyme, which means we can no longer digest the milk sugar lactose. Consuming lactose without the lactase enzyme can lead to symptoms such as abdominal bloating, gas, cramping, and diarrhea. It can also decrease the body's ability to absorb thyroid medications.

The proteins casein and whey can cause food sensitivities, creating specific types of immune responses. These anecdotally have been shown to increase antibodies against the thyroid and increase brain fog.

Soy

Soy is an inexpensive protein found in soybeans that is often used as a filler in many foods. The problem with soy is that it is a xenoestrogen, which means that the body can mistake it for the hormone estrogen. The excess of estrogen, or what looks like estrogen, can be a trigger for an immune response in people with Hashimoto's.

Soy is also a goitrogen, which is a substance that can interfere with the thyroid's ability to produce thyroid hormones. While goitrogens are found in many foods, soy is particularly high in goitrogen and has more of a negative impact on the thyroid.

Caffeine, Sugar, and Alcohol

Caffeine, sugar, and alcohol work similarly to cause stress by increasing cortisol production and creating blood sugar instability. They all produce large swings in the adrenal gland's production of cortisol. This swing in cortisol production releases inflammatory proteins, causing low-grade systemic inflammation in the body. These also individually cause blood sugar dysregulation, creating swings in blood sugar that the body perceives as stress, which ultimately produces inflammation.

FAQs

When it comes to your role in managing Hashimoto's, there are many factors to consider. Here are a few of the most common questions I've heard as a practitioner, and answers to help you better understand your disease.

What is a goiter and how does it affect Hashimoto's?

A goiter is the term used when the thyroid gland is abnormally enlarged. It can occur when a gland is producing too much, too little, or the appropriate amount of thyroid hormone, or with the immune system involvement of Hashimoto's. In the case of Hashimoto's, as the thyroid gland sustains more damage, it creates a higher demand on the thyroid to produce more hormone. The overstimulation of the thyroid can result in a goiter.

I heard that I should not eat healthy vegetables like broccoli because they have goitrogens. What are goitrogens and is that true?

A goitrogen is a substance found in some medications, foods, and chemicals that can interrupt the way the thyroid uses iodine to make hormones. Goitrogens are found in foods such as soy, cassava, broccoli, cabbage, kale, spinach, cauliflower, bok choy, and Brussels sprouts. Not all goitrogens in these foods have the same goitrogenic effects. Many vegetables that contain goitrogens also contain a variety of vitamins, minerals, and phytochemicals that are beneficial. Cooking these vegetables also greatly decreases the impact of the goitrogens. When taken with appropriate doses of iodine, these foods (with the exception of soy, as it is well-established to be an endocrine disruptor) can be a healthy addition to the diet.

Can I be a vegetarian or vegan and still manage Hashimoto's?

Creating a well-balanced, nutrient-dense vegetarian or vegan diet takes a significant amount of dedication. It has been my experience that many of the foods consumed on a vegetarian or vegan diet are not ideal for providing the proper nutrient and hormone balance needed for managing Hashimoto's, specifically when going through an elimination diet. That said, plant-based, nutrient-rich foods are an integral part of managing Hashimoto's.

Can I lose weight with Hashimoto's?

There are many reasons why it's hard to lose weight with a Hashimoto's diagnosis. Since the thyroid is the primary controller of the metabolism, it is critical to get these hormones regulated and low-grade inflammation reduced before weight loss will occur. Not only is it important for thyroid hormones to be regulated, but the insulin and reproductive hormones also play a role in weight gain and must be balanced.

What's the difference between a food allergy and a food sensitivity?

The difference between a food allergy and a food sensitivity is how much the immune system is involved. Immunoglobulins are proteins produced by the immune system to destroy foreign substances. There are five levels of immunoglobulins—IgA, IgG, IgM, IgD, and IgE. When an attack escalates to the IgE level, it is considered an allergy and usually results in immediate reactions. Food sensitivities can be delayed for as long as three days, and involve the immune system by creating IgG and IgA immunoglobulins. While sensitivities are not life-threatening, the constant immune response can still be damaging to the body.

Nutrition and the Thyroid

As with any organ, there are specific nutrients that are essential to optimal thyroid function. Designing your diet to include these nutrients is ideal; however, sometimes supplementation can be critical to help you feel better quickly. When you feel better, you have the energy to get through the day, clearly think through your foggy brain, and make better decisions for yourself.

Tyrosine, Iodine, and Iron

The thyroid uses tyrosine, iodine, and iron in building the T4 hormone. Tyrosine is found in a large variety of foods, including high-protein foods such as chicken and turkey, as well as bananas, peanuts, and avocado. An insufficiency is very rare.

Iodine is found primarily in foods that come from the sea—fish, shrimp, and sea vegetables such as kelp, nori, and kombu—which is not common dinner fare for most people. Supplementation with iodine can be useful for those with

Hashimoto's; however, it has a specific range where it is advantageous. Excessive iodine can be as detrimental as a deficiency. If you're supplementing, a dose no higher than 200mcg per day is recommended.

Iron, also used in hormone production, is commonly found in red meats, organ meats, and dark leafy greens. However, if someone has gastrointestinal issues, inability to absorb nutrients, or has been following a vegetarian diet, they may not be getting enough iron. A simple lab test of iron and ferritin (the storage form of iron) can be requested from your medical team. If needed, it can be supplemented with as much as 20mg to 45mg per day.

Zinc and Selenium

Zinc and selenium are needed to convert T4 into usable T3. The highest amounts of zinc are found in oysters, red meat, and pumpkin seeds. Selenium is highest in Brazil nuts but is also found in meats and seafood. Both are crucial to healthy hormone function. These can also be supplemented with 30mg to 45mg of zinc and 200mcg to 400mcg of selenium per day.

The B Vitamins

Other nutrients that are useful for the proper function of your thyroid hormones are B vitamins (there are eight), including B6 and B12, which provide the body with energy. This is done by converting calories, through a series of complex chemical reactions, into the specific form of energy the cells use, called ATP. These nutrients can be obtained from foods high in B vitamins, such as leafy greens and legumes, or can be taken in a vitamin B complex supplement.

An additional 600mg of B1 (thiamin) may be beneficial if you are feeling particularly sluggish. Thiamin, found in beef, liver, nuts, eggs, and legumes, is useful for converting carbohydrates into energy; thus it is also useful for preventing fatigue. Two of the less commonly known but essential B vitamins are B2 (riboflavin) and B3 (niacin). They can be found in a variety of foods, including eggs, meats, and green vegetables, and are needed for the development of T4. While you can get these nutrients from foods, you may choose to supplement with a general vitamin B complex.

Magnesium and Vitamins D, A, and C

Some nutrients are used in smaller amounts but are vital for thyroid function and its supporting organs. Magnesium is a mineral that is used for 300 different functions in the body. It is essential for supporting the liver, which is the primary organ used in the conversion of T4 to T3. Magnesium is also crucial for adrenal health, which is a sister gland to the thyroid. Magnesium is found in foods such as nuts, seeds, and green leafy vegetables. However, if you want to supplement, 200mg to 400mg of magnesium glycinate is a good place to start.

Vitamin D acts as a communicator in the body and is necessary for producing hormones. There are a few foods that contain vitamin D, such as salmon, egg yolks, and mushrooms; however, our best source of vitamin D is the sun, where the skin converts sunlight to the usable form of vitamin D. Since most of us don't get enough sun exposure throughout the year, supplementing with 2,000IUs to 5,000IUs is a good dose to keep your vitamin D in the optimal range.

There are two main forms of vitamin A that help improve how each cell in the body uses thyroid hormones. Vitamin A is found in orange foods such as carrots, sweet potatoes, and orange bell peppers, and also in dark leafy greens and egg yolks. Vitamin A supplementation is best found in a general multivitamin.

Vitamin C contributes to the production of thyroid hormones. It's commonly known to be found in citrus foods, but broccoli, bell peppers, and Brussels sprouts are also very high in vitamin C. If you are not eating these foods regularly, supplementation with 500mg to 3,000mg daily can be beneficial. Vitamin C is a water-soluble vitamin, so your body will only use what it needs and eliminate the rest in your urine.

The Power of an Elimination Diet

Food is a powerful tool. It can be used to support your body, or your food choices can work against you. Everyone has a diet that works best for them, and it is as unique as your fingerprint. The challenge is identifying what works best for you, which is exactly what you will uncover throughout this process.

Our food industry spends a significant amount of time and money focusing on creating products with the perfect combination of fat, sugar, and salt to make our foods super-palatable. While they may taste good momentarily, these foods do not support our bodies in functioning at the highest level. And many of these common foods create low-grade inflammation, which can result in symptoms such as headaches, joint pain, bloating, and fatigue, and eventually lead to an autoimmune response.

An elimination diet is a multipronged approach to healing. The diet protocol laid out in this book eliminates common trigger foods—gluten, dairy, soy, sugar, caffeine, and alcohol—to decrease both inflammation and autoimmune response. It will also support the thyroid's sister glands, the adrenals, by balancing cortisol, which will affect immune function. In addition, an elimination diet aids in balancing blood sugar and the hormone insulin. Since these hormones work synergistically when they are all supported, they will be able to balance themselves. Finally, this diet incorporates the foods that have the key nutrients necessary to support thyroid function.

Potential trigger foods are removed for 21 days, allowing the gastrointestinal and immune systems to calm and balance themselves. In many cases, symptoms you may have been dealing with for a long time will subside, such as joint pain, bloating, bowel upset, fatigue, and poor sleep quality—all probable signs of inflammation. Consider this a healing diet for your gastrointestinal tract and your thyroid. After the elimination phase, slowly reintroducing foods and tracking your symptoms will allow you to create your customized diet.

During the reintroduction phase you will introduce one food at a time, then evaluate how your body reacts. When reintroducing foods, you will first add a food back into your diet, then document any symptoms. Since symptoms can sometimes take as long as three days to surface, you will introduce only one new food every four days. With careful notes and documentation, you will learn which foods you want to permanently remove from your diet and which ones make you feel your best, thus creating your personalized diet.

The Doctor Is In

As with any diagnosis, there are many questions that arise about Hashimoto's. Here are some of the top questions to ask your doctor or health care practitioner, as well as common answers you may hear to these questions.

How often do my labs need to be drawn and medications adjusted?

For most Hashimoto's patients, after they start taking medication, the dose can be adjusted every six to eight weeks until thyroid hormone labs are normal and symptoms have resolved. Once they're on a maintenance dose, the labs can be drawn every six to twelve months, adjusting as needed. However, if symptoms arise it may be necessary to monitor more frequently. Consult with your doctor to determine how often you should consider coming in for routine lab work and a medication evaluation.

How do I know if the medication is working or if I need to adjust it?

There are many medications that can be used as part of the treatment for Hashimoto's, some with only T4 hormone, some with only T3 hormone, and some with both. When you start a medication, it takes about four to six weeks for your body to adapt to the additional hormones. If your symptoms persist after six to eight weeks, it may mean that your medication dose needs to be adjusted, providing more or less of the hormone, or a different hormone combination. Speak to your doctor.

Will I always need to be on medications for my thyroid?

In the case of Hashimoto's (as opposed to hypothyroidism), when there is an immune response it's unlikely that your thyroid will be able to produce enough hormones on its own. This means medications will likely always be one of the tools used to support the hormone your thyroid is making, to ensure that you have adequate thyroid hormones.

Do I need to have a thyroid ultrasound?

A thyroid ultrasound is useful for identifying nodules and goiters. If your doctor recognizes a nodule or goiter by feeling your neck, they may order an ultrasound to further evaluate it. Additionally, if your doctor suspects Hashimoto's but your labs don't show antibodies, an ultrasound may be warranted. Ultimately, an ultrasound is a way to evaluate the thyroid to determine how much damage has occurred within it.

(continued on next page)

What are nodules and do they affect my thyroid function?

A thyroid nodule is a growth of thyroid cells that create a lump in the thyroid. Nodules can be filled with fluid or can be solid. They form individually or in clusters. Nodules are very common and are thought to be related to iodine deficiency. While over 90 percent of thyroid nodules are non-cancerous, if there is any question, the nodule can be biopsied for evaluation.

Build a Support System

The road to healing can be a long and winding one, so you will need to build a support team around you. Your team has many players, all with specific roles. While you are the captain, your team is there to help guide you and assist in troubleshooting any issues that arise during your healing process.

Your Health Care Team

Because you received a Hashimoto's diagnosis, it's safe to assume you have a pretty solid team of health care practitioners behind you helping you manage your disease. These are the people who will help translate and treat your symptoms, prescribe and adjust your medications and other treatments, and be with you every step of the way to answer your questions and provide professional feedback as you navigate your diagnosis.

Physician: Whether a general practitioner or an endocrinologist, your doctor has the role of listening, educating, and supervising your healing process. They will be the one who prescribes and manages your medications. They should be open-minded and supportive.

Registered dietitian or nutritionist: This is the person who will help instruct you on new foods, recipes, and nutrients that you can incorporate into your diet. They are there to listen and help you troubleshoot what foods are working and what foods are not working for you.

Health coach: A health coach can motivate and cheerlead you throughout your journey.

Your Social Circle

The rest of your support team consists of people you lean on when you need encouragement. These can include a therapist, a coach, friends who will lend an ear, and your family members.

Although we know Hashimoto's can make you feel lousy on the inside, your outside body may not always appear to be in distress. This can make it difficult for people who are not going through the process to understand it, because you don't look different. It's important to have the right words to explain it, and I encourage you to keep your explanation simple and to the point. Inform them that you are taking an active role in your healing process. It could sound something like this: *My thyroid is having trouble regulating itself. As a result, I feel tired and uncomfortable sometimes, even though I don't look any different. I am working with my medical team to take the right steps to start the healing process and feel better. I need your support to help me through this process.*

Most people are willing to support you but they don't exactly know how. It's crucial that you tell them exactly what you need from them. In some cases, you may need help with your children, such as cooking them dinner or driving them to various activities. Sometimes you may need help with keeping the house tidy. Be specific, because what your family member may consider helpful may not necessarily be useful to you. For example: *You can support me by . . .*

- *cooking dinner one night a week.*
- *carpooling the kids to school.*
- *eating your unhealthy foods when I'm not around, so I'm not tempted.*

When it comes to preparing for the elimination diet, you will also need buy-in from the people closest to you. Ask them to be a part of the diet with you, because it's easier with a group or an accountability partner. Remind them that this is a short time period; it's not forever, and it will likely help them feel good, too!

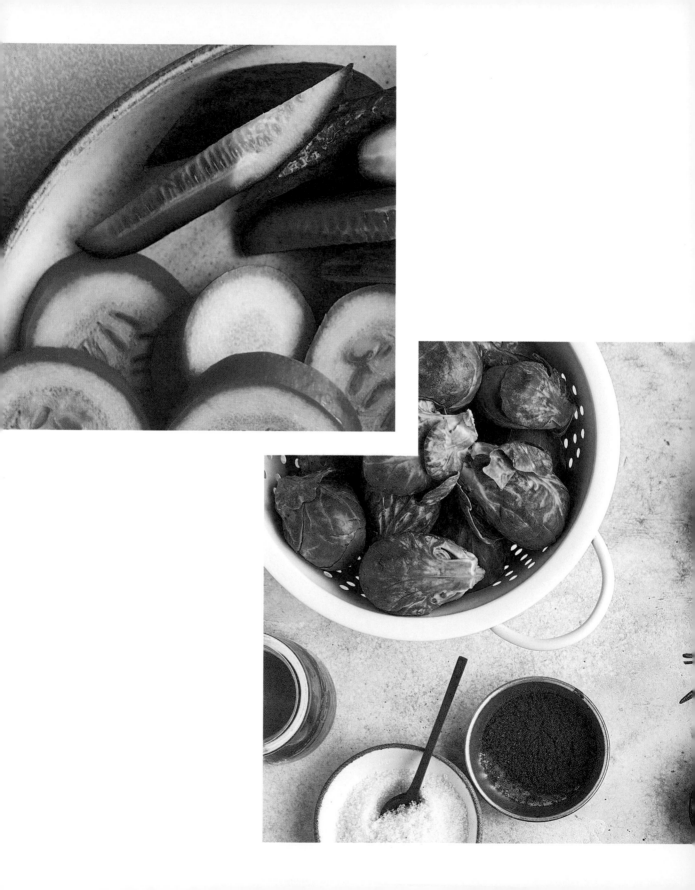

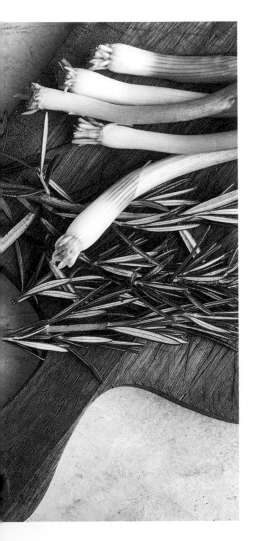

CHAPTER 2

Getting Ready for the Elimination Diet

While healing from Hashimoto's requires a multifaceted approach, feeding yourself is one aspect of life that you have the most control over. An elimination diet is a powerful tool that can help you determine which foods will work best for you to live as symptom-free and pain-free as possible. It is the critical first step to moving forward.

This diet plan requires motivation and commitment. It takes planning, persistence, and hard work for 21 days. It will help you build sustainable healing habits, as well as develop an understanding of what's working and not working in your body. You must be patient, as this is a marathon, not a sprint. In all honesty, you may feel worse for a few days before feeling better—but hang in there. This is your body's way of flushing out your system and then flooding it with the nutrients that will support you.

And remember, this 21-day elimination is only temporary, and this book will help and support you every step of the way. This is a temporary means to an end and, when done correctly, it can set you on the path of healing for an enjoyable and symptom-free life.

How to Do the Elimination Diet

This next section will set you up with everything you need to know as you start on this critical step down your path to healing. We've done all the hard work—planning meals, making shopping lists, figuring out recipes—to minimize the stress on you.

What to Eat

Despite its name, the elimination diet is not just a list of foods you *can't* eat. In fact, let's start with the long list of delicious, nutrient-dense foods you'll be encouraged to consume over the next 21 days, and beyond.

Fruits: Fruits are full of vitamins and minerals, and their rich colors provide important phytochemicals. Blueberries, blackberries, strawberries, raspberries, grapefruit, oranges, cherries, apples, plums, and pears are all great fruits that provide nutrients but do not cause large fluctuations in blood sugar. They can be eaten as part of a snack or mixed into your meals.

Vegetables: Also known for their nutrient density, vegetables are a good source of fiber, which works well for blood sugar management. In addition, vegetables such as broccoli, cabbage, Brussels sprouts, cauliflower, spinach, kale, Swiss chard, and other leafy greens are beneficial for estrogen metabolism. This is helpful for supporting the thyroid hormones to work efficiently.

Starchy root vegetables and winter squash: Root veggies are usually starchier, which means that they have more carbohydrates than their non-starchy counterparts. While they have more carbs, they are also nutrient-dense and provide many of the nutrients needed to support thyroid and adrenal hormone production. These veggies include sweet potatoes, carrots, beets, turnips, butternut squash, and acorn squash.

Healthy fats: Fats are necessary for a healthy diet. The ones most advantageous for this diet are found in pumpkin seeds, sunflower seeds, Brazil nuts, almonds, avocados, egg yolks, coconut products, and olives. Not only can these fats calm an inflammatory response, but they are also a great source of zinc, selenium, fiber, and tyrosine.

Meats and seafood: In their whole forms, animal proteins provide critical amino acids and iodine. They are also a rich source of tyrosine, zinc, and iron, all necessary for building thyroid hormones. In their whole, unprocessed forms, meats, such as chicken, turkey, beef, lamb, organ meats, fish, oysters, shrimp, salmon, and broths will not only keep you full, but also provide protein to aid in the healing process.

Non-glutenous grains: In this elimination diet, we stick to grains that do not contain gluten and do not have a significant impact on blood sugar. These grains are a source of fiber and a variety of vitamins and minerals. The non-glutenous grains include amaranth, quinoa, gluten-free oats, buckwheat, sorghum, and corn. You may notice that rice is not listed. Although gluten-free, both brown and white rice cause blood sugar elevations that we want to avoid.

Flavor enhancers: Other flavor enhancers are useful not only for providing flavor to foods, but also in the healing process. These include cilantro, rosemary, thyme, oregano, and other herbs and spices. Sea salt and Himalayan salt are recommended because they are naturally rich in minerals that are stripped out in commercial table salt.

Sweeteners: The primary issue with sweeteners is the impact they have on blood glucose levels. In small amounts, natural sweeteners such as honey and maple syrup can be used. Other sweeteners that have minimal impact on blood sugar but aren't chemical in nature include monk fruit, erythritol, and stevia.

What to Eliminate

This elimination diet is not only the first step on your path to healing; you can also consider it a training process to eat nutrient-dense foods for a lifetime. The nutrition you find in wholesome, real foods will help you feel better and prevent further chronic diseases. This means saying goodbye to some trigger foods that may have become staples for you—foods that aren't supportive of healthy functioning.

Gluten: This includes bread and bread-type products (biscuits, waffles, pancakes, flour tortillas), crackers, pasta, cereals, cookies, cakes, and pastries. These traditionally gluten-filled foods can, in many cases, be found in a gluten-free version; however, even the gluten-free versions of these foods are highly processed and stripped of most nutritional value. To support the health of your immune system, they will need to be permanently eliminated from your diet for optimal results and healing.

Processed foods: Foods such as chips, doughnuts, granola bars, microwave popcorn, instant meals such as ramen or macaroni and cheese, and anything fried or battered not only have minimal nutritional value, but are also loaded with additives and preservatives that can be detrimental to how your body functions.

High-sugar foods and beverages: Candy, jelly, syrup, sodas, sports drinks, and fruit juices will wreak havoc on your blood sugar and insulin levels. They are highly processed, which strips them of any of the B vitamins that are found in natural sugar. Additionally, foods and beverages with sugar—both white sugar and brown sugar, and even naturally and minimally processed sugars—cause significant blood sugar fluctuations that should be avoided.

Sugar substitutes: Also recognizable as the pink, blue, and yellow packs of saccharin, aspartame, and sucralose, sugar substitutes are found in many diet and sugar-free foods and drinks. While they don't have the carbohydrates that will affect blood sugar, they can affect your cravings for sugar and other high-carbohydrate foods and can have long-term neurological effects.

What to Avoid Temporarily

There is no cure for Hashimoto's, but you can play a big role in managing your symptoms and supporting the organs that work together with the thyroid. This elimination diet is designed for the person who is just starting to work with food to manage their Hashimoto's symptoms. It starts by eliminating the foods that are most likely to cause inflammation. While some foods in the standard American diet need to be completely eliminated for good, everyone's tolerance for certain foods is highly individualized, so you may be able to reintroduce some foods. The whole idea behind an elimination diet is to determine what foods you need to avoid permanently, what foods can be reintroduced in smaller amounts, and what foods work well for you.

Since this process is new for you, this diet is a beginner's approach. The elimination is not as strict as a complete autoimmune protocol, because we are focused on making this easy to implement and getting you good results so you can feel better fast.

This diet is a first step toward eliminating the "big players." Once you get through this initial phase, if your symptoms have not improved you may need to move on to the Next-Level Elimination (see page 24).

As I have already mentioned, foods that include gluten, sugar, or sugar substitutes, and any processed foods must be totally eliminated. However, there are some other foods that, while you may be able to tolerate them, should also be eliminated for the 21-day period. After the elimination period, you can slowly reintroduce them, and may even find that they do not affect your Hashimoto's.

Soy: Known as an endocrine disruptor, soy can be problematic for many hormones in the endocrine system. As it relates to the thyroid, soy can block the enzymatic process of converting T4 into T3.

Caffeine and alcohol: Caffeine and alcohol affect blood sugar balance and adrenal function. The adrenal glands are the sister glands of the thyroid, and when the thyroid is not functioning at its best it will affect the functioning of the adrenals. To balance the thyroid hormones you have to support adrenals. Keeping blood sugar balanced throughout the day allows the adrenals to stabilize. Eliminating caffeine and alcohol will help with that.

Dairy: There are three components to dairy that are often problematic: Lactose is the sugar in dairy, and casein and whey are two types of proteins. Lactose may cause abdominal bloating and discomfort. The proteins can cause an increased immune response for someone who has intestinal permeability, also known as leaky gut. Based on the work of Dr. Alessio Fasano, intestinal permeability is a precursor to developing an autoimmune disease.

If you find yourself 14 days into the elimination diet and you are still not feeling better, there are a few other foods that could potentially be impeding your healing process. These are what I'm calling "Next-Level Elimination" foods. They are included in some of the recipes in the second part of this book because they do not trigger symptoms for everyone with Hashimoto's—but they do trigger symptoms for some. (Remember, we said that everyone's tolerance for particular foods is highly individualized.) If you find yourself still experiencing symptoms, you may need to eliminate these foods.

Eggs: While eggs are a good source of nutrition, some egg white proteins can permeate the intestinal barrier, causing an already hyperactive immune system to react even more. It is possible that eliminating eggs in all forms may be necessary to decrease your immune response.

Nightshades: Nightshades are a class of foods that have a natural chemical in them called solanine. For some, solanine is related to inflammation, which is reflected in joint pain, acid reflux, or skin rashes. Foods that fall into the family of nightshades include tomatoes, eggplant, all kinds of peppers and pepper spices, and white potatoes. (Sweet potatoes are not in the same family.) White potatoes also tend to spike blood sugar, so either eliminate them or use them very sparingly.

Grains: While glutenous grains are likely to cause an autoimmune response, for some people all grains can be problematic. These include even the non-gluten ones such as oats, rice, corn, quinoa, and less common grains such as buckwheat and millet. This also means eliminating grain-based milks such as oat milk and rice milk.

Nuts and seeds: All nuts and seeds may be problematic. This includes almonds, cashews, Brazil nuts, walnuts, pecans, and the nut butters that are made from them; and all seeds, such as sunflower seeds, sesame seeds, chia seeds, hemp seeds; and seed butters such as tahini and sunflower butter. You should also eliminate nut-based and seed-based milks, such as almond, cashew, and hemp milk. Coconut milk, however, is always allowed unless you know that you have a reaction to coconut.

Beans and legumes: Due to the lectins (proteins that bind to carbohydrates), all beans and legumes may be potential triggers. This includes lentils, black beans, white beans, red or kidney beans, garbanzo beans—even hummus. In addition, peas such as green peas, field peas, and black-eyed peas can potentially trigger an immune response.

Onions and garlic: While onions and garlic don't cause an immune response, some people find them to be difficult on their bellies. They can potentially cause gas, bloating, and abdominal discomfort. If you experience these, you might try a trial elimination of onions, garlic, and their powders.

Several recipes in this book are labeled as "Next-Level Elimination–friendly," which means that they are free of all foods that may cause symptoms—not just the first-level elimination foods outlined in this chapter. However, for many other recipes I've included Next-Level Elimination tips for removing or replacing these next-level elimination ingredients whenever possible. If a recipe just can't work without eggs, and you find that they are one of your trigger foods, just skip that recipe. There are more than 70 recipes in this book, so I promise there is still plenty for you to eat!

Mind Your Mindset

As with any habit or lifestyle change, the initial transition to an elimination diet can be difficult. The first step in a successful elimination diet is changing your mindset. A few tips:

- Go into this with a positive outlook, knowing that you have absolutely everything you need to get through it. Yes, you will be giving up some foods you love. But you will also be taking active steps to feel healthier and more alert and energetic. You have everything to gain. Remember: This elimination diet is temporary.

- Assess what you have in your kitchen and pantry, and remove anything that will not play a supportive role in your journey, making room for the foods that will help you begin your healing process.

- Once your headspace is clear and your kitchen is ready, set a date and begin. Make a serious commitment, and make time for what that commitment entails. Look over your calendar for the next 21 days and identify times when you can plan, shop, and prepare foods. If this is not what you typically do, it may feel like a huge time commitment, but it is absolutely necessary to help you manage the diet. You will get better and faster at this, and it will get easier.

When you start the diet there is a possibility that you may feel worse before you feel better. It's unfortunate, but it is true. This is very common, as your body is starting to let go of things that it's been holding on to that don't serve it—mainly dietary toxins. If there are a lot of toxins you may feel tired, fatigued, and more sluggish, but don't give up. As your body clears these toxins, you *will* start to feel better. You are the little engine that could, so keep moving forward.

Prep Your Kitchen

As with any new process, preparation is your key to success. This section will help you set up your kitchen—from food to appliances—to ease the transition and follow the elimination diet outlined in this book. First, let's discuss what Hashimoto's-friendly ingredients and foods to stock up on in your pantry, spice rack, freezer, and refrigerator. Then we'll go over the kitchen tools and appliances necessary for success with the recipes in Part 2.

Pantry and Spice Rack

When cleaning out your pantry, you will likely find foods we've already listed as eliminated from the diet. Donate them to a food pantry, throw them out, or put them somewhere out of sight in the back of the cabinet (for entertaining or when cooking for others).

When deciding what to keep and what to toss, read the ingredients list on the labels and look for problematic ingredients such as sugar, wheat, flour, or gluten. Some unexpected places you might find flour include taco seasoning or chili seasoning packets. Sugar hides in many places also, such as in ketchup, BBQ sauce, marinades, and salad dressings. Used in small amounts, they can be okay, but use them with great caution so you don't affect your blood sugar.

Now that you've cleared some space in your pantry and spice rack, let's stock them for success for the elimination diet and after. Following are the ingredients you'll need for the elimination diet outlined in this book. However, if you are not feeling better after the first 14 days and want to do a deeper Next-Level Elimination, remove the ingredients that I've noted with an asterisk.

Pantry

- Apple cider vinegar
- Arrowroot powder
- Balsamic vinegar
- Beans* and lentils*
- Broth: chicken, beef, and/or vegetable
- Cocoa powder*
- Coconut aminos (soy sauce replacement)
- Coconut milk, full-fat canned
- Grains*: amaranth, quinoa, and corn
- Herbal teas
- Nuts* and nut butters*
- Oils: avocado, coconut, and extra-virgin olive
- Seeds* and seed butters*

Herbs and Spices

- Bay leaves
- Cardamom, ground
- Celery leaves, dried
- Chili powder*
- Cinnamon, ground and whole sticks
- Coriander, ground
- Cumin, ground*
- Dill, dried
- Garlic powder**
- Ginger, ground
- Nutmeg, ground*
- Onion powder**
- Oregano, dried

- Paprika, dried*
- Pepper*, ground or whole peppercorns
- Salt, preferably sea salt or Himalayan salt
- Spice blends
- Thyme, dried
- Turmeric, ground
- Vanilla extract

*If your symptoms do not subside, eliminate these foods for Next-Level Elimination.
**If gas and bloating are problematic, try eliminating onion and garlic.

Refrigerator and Freezer

Rummage through the refrigerator and freezer to clear out everything that will not support your journey to health and wellness. If you choose to keep foods that you should eliminate or avoid in order to use them when cooking for your family or entertaining, be sure to separate and clearly mark which foods work for you and which don't, so you're not tempted to reach for eliminated foods or use them accidentally.

Be aware that many frozen, prepared meals sold in the grocery stores are full of additives and preservatives and should be avoided on a Hashimoto's-friendly diet. Keep this in mind when shopping. We all like to be able to grab things from the refrigerator or freezer and pop them in the oven or microwave, and you can on this diet, too. Simply double many of the recipes in this book and freeze them for future quick and easy meals. You'll find storage, freezing, and reheating instructions for most of them right in the recipe.

Fill your refrigerator and/or freezer with the following foods for success. As with the pantry items, if you are not feeling better after the first 14 days and want to do a deeper Next-Level Elimination, remove the ingredients that I've noted with an asterisk.

Meat, Poultry, and Seafood

Any cuts of unprocessed chicken, turkey, beef, or lamb, and any type of fish or shellfish are fine on your diet. Buying grass-fed, pastured, wild, or organic is ideal; however, choose the best quality you can afford. You can buy proteins in bulk and store them in the freezer to use later, or buy them already frozen. Well-wrapped and sealed chicken, turkey, beef, and lamb will keep in the freezer for six to twelve months. Well-wrapped and sealed fish and shellfish maintain their quality for up six months in the freezer.

Fruits and Vegetables

Fresh produce is great; frozen is also fine. In fact, frozen produce can be more nutrient-rich than fresh because it's picked and frozen at its ripest, preserving the nutritional value. It's best to include both fresh and frozen on your grocery list, based on your shopping and cooking schedule. Organic is always ideal to avoid the chemicals from pesticides and fertilizers; however, buy the best quality produce you can afford.

Fruits: Apples, avocados, bananas, berries (blackberries, blueberries, raspberries, strawberries), cherries, dates, grapes, melons, nectarines, papayas, peaches, pears, plums, pomegranates

Vegetables: Artichokes, asparagus, beets, bok choy, broccoli, Brussels sprouts, cabbage, carrots, cauliflower, celery, cucumber, fennel, garlic**, ginger, green beans, greens (beet, chard, collards, mustard), kale, lettuce (all varieties), mushrooms, onions**, parsley, parsnips, peas, spinach, squashes (all varieties), sweet potatoes and yams, turnips, zucchini

Other Goodies

There are many other staples that it will be helpful to have stocked in your refrigerator. These include condiments, dressings, dairy-free milk, and nut and seed butters. Some of these may need to be eliminated if you move to the Next-Level Elimination plan (I've marked those with an asterisk), but give them a try for the initial elimination diet.

You will find recipes and storage instructions for some of these staples (and others) in chapter 10. The idea is to make them on the weekends, and then just pull the jar out of the refrigerator and use it as conveniently as if it were store-bought. You'll also find suggestions in that chapter for choosing store-bought brands. There are now a variety of brands of foods like salad dressings and mayonnaise that are Hashimoto's-friendly, some of which are turning up in regular grocery stores and almost all of which can be purchased online.

- Eggs*
- Dairy-free milk: unsweetened coconut milk, oat milk*, almond milk*, and cashew milk*
- Nut* and seed butters*
- Yellow and Dijon mustard
- Fermented veggies: sauerkraut, kimchi, and fermented pickles
- Ghee (the fat from butter with the dairy solids removed)
- Salad dressings made without soybean oil, store-bought or homemade
- Mayonnaise made without soybean oil, store-bought or homemade
- Olives

*If your symptoms do not subside, eliminate these foods for Next-Level Elimination.
**If gas and bloating are problematic, try eliminating onion and garlic.

Appliances and Kitchen Tools

To make this process even easier, I've listed the appliances and tools you'll need to be successful in the kitchen. In general, aim for tools that are made of glass, wood, or stainless steel, as these are non-toxic (unlike plastic materials). It's best to avoid using nonstick pans—especially Teflon pans—as they can be hazardous for your thyroid because they leach chemicals and metals into your food.

Must-Have

- Stainless steel measuring spoons and cups
- Large stainless steel, bamboo, or wooden spoons and spatulas
- Wooden or silicone cutting board(s)
- Parchment paper (for nonstick baking)
- Good quality, sharp knives
- Glass or stainless-steel storage containers in different sizes (plastic lids are okay)
- Wide-mouth glass jars with lids

- High-powered blender
- Food processor
- Stainless steel colander
- Baking sheets
- Glass or ceramic baking dishes
- 10-inch or 12-inch stainless steel or cast iron skillet
- 2-quart stainless steel pot with lid
- 8 quart (or bigger) stainless steel pot with lid

Nice to Have

Because the following appliances and tools are not listed as must-haves, I've included explanations for why you might consider adding them to your kitchen.

Stainless steel immersion blender: great for creating quick sauces or smoothies if you don't want to pull out the standing blender

Garlic press: makes adding the aromatic flavors and antimicrobial properties of garlic much easier

Electric pressure cooker: allows for quick and nearly effortless meals

Slow cooker: great for long cooking times without much effort

Toaster oven: ideal for reheating leftovers

Air fryer: gives you the crisp of fried foods without the oils that go along with them

Shop and Chop

Now that your kitchen is ready, it's time to conquer the grocery store and learn how to streamline meal preparation.

Navigating the Grocery Store

By this point you should have looked at your calendar and identified "day one" of the elimination diet. Your next step is to create a plan for week one. Plan for only one week at a time—this keeps your plan manageable and not overwhelming. To make this as easy as possible, I've included meal plans for each week of the elimination diet in the next chapter, as well as weekly shopping lists.

Speaking of shopping, let's tackle your first trip to the grocery store. You may be navigating parts of the grocery store that are unfamiliar to you, so go armed with your list and a little extra time. Here are a few of my tips and tricks for making your grocery shopping trips easy, manageable, and stress-free.

Shop for the best food quality that you can get. Some words to look for include *organic, non-GMO, antibiotic-free, wild, sustainably caught, grass-fed,* and *pastured.* Don't stress about making everything perfect; just do the best you can within these parameters. And remember, only buy what fits your budget.

Shop the perimeter. The grocery store is set up to have the best quality, freshest foods around the perimeter of the store: Fresh fruits and vegetables are usually in the front, fresh meats are along the side, and frozen vegetables are usually in the back. Stay in these areas as much as possible to limit the temptation of purchasing processed or packaged foods, and to keep your shopping experience short and sweet.

Your first trip to the grocery store may be more expensive, but don't fret. You will be buying staples such as oils, broths, and flours that will last throughout the diet, so you won't have to buy these every week. You can also save money by finding the self-serve bulk section and buying only what you need.

Shop for groceries online. The food industry has realized that there is a need for clean foods that are different from the processed, salty, artificially flavored foods our grandmothers bought. Sometimes these foods are not in conventional supermarkets. You don't have to run all over town to health food and specialty stores; just shop online. Some products that may be easier to find online include raw nuts and seeds, coconut aminos, Asian fish sauce, arrowroot, monk fruit sweeteners, and nutritional yeast. Some of the cleaner brands of salad dressing, mayonnaise, and other sauces may also be easier to get online. In fact, you could do all your grocery shopping online if that works better for you. You can shop when and where you want, even dressed in your jammies, and everything is delivered directly to your door. This can also be helpful if the supermarket is full of too many temptations for you.

Mastering Meal Prep

The meal prepping process is an essential part of your plan. Here are a few tips to help make you a meal prep master—and to make preparation as easy as possible.

When you can, buy fruits and veggies already sliced and diced. You can buy things such as riced cauliflower, spiralized zucchini, diced onions, and shredded Brussels sprouts. This is one less step for you to do at home.

Break up your shopping and meal prep days to make it easier for you. For example, you can buy groceries on one day, then spend some time the next day prepping and storing things for quick use later. That makes the actual cooking day much easier.

Roast lots of veggies at one time, using different baking sheets. Whenever you're using the oven, cook multiple foods and store some for later. You can roast beets and cauliflower at the same time. You can also bake sweet potatoes that can be frozen whole for later use.

Always have a protein cooked and ready to go. Whether it's in the refrigerator or freezer, always have something that is already prepared. This can be anything from diced chicken thighs to cooked turkey burgers. Having something on hand ensures you won't deviate from the plan just for the sake of convenience.

If you are preparing meals for others, ask for help. There's no shame in asking your children, spouse, or roommate to wash fruit or chop vegetables, especially if you are preparing meals for them.

Keep your staples on hand. Some staple foods are essential for keeping the meal prep process moving smoothly. These include cauliflower rice, baked sweet potatoes, salad dressings, and sauces to spruce up some meals. Having these always prepared makes meals much easier. (You'll find recipes for all of them in chapter 10.)

Succeeding on an Elimination Diet

Everyone has a diet that works for them; that's what this book is helping you fine-tune. There are some common challenges that people face on this journey, including using the elimination diet as a weight-loss diet, slipping up, and discovering unexpected sensitivities. Here are some tips for dealing with these challenges.

A Note on Weight Loss

The purpose of the elimination diet is to discover what foods work for you and what foods do not. Although you may lose weight, this is not a weight-loss diet so there is no need to skimp on your meals. You are not counting calories or weighing foods. While many diets ask you to monitor the amount of food you eat, this elimination diet is based on the quality of food, not the quantity. Eat when you are hungry, and until you are satisfied.

Overcoming Slip-Ups

You aren't perfect, so you may slip up and eat something you should be eliminating. This happens by accident in many cases, as you find a hidden ingredient in something you forgot to read the label on. Or you might not plan well and find yourself famished and looking for anything you can get your hands on. Either way, use it as a learning opportunity. First, figure out why you slipped up. Then, pay attention to how you feel afterward. Depending on how far you are into the process, you may find that you feel the effect of the offending food—as we'll talk about in chapter 4 on how to reintroduce foods and track your symptoms.

Uncovering Unexpected Food Sensitivities

It is possible that you are sensitive to foods that are listed as "allowed" on the elimination diet. For instance, while coconut products are a healthy fat, some people have a sensitivity to coconut. If you find a food that doesn't make you feel well, causes skin irritation, or creates loose stools, add it to your list of foods to temporarily eliminate, pick another recipe for your meal plan, and test the offending food again later during the reintroduction phase.

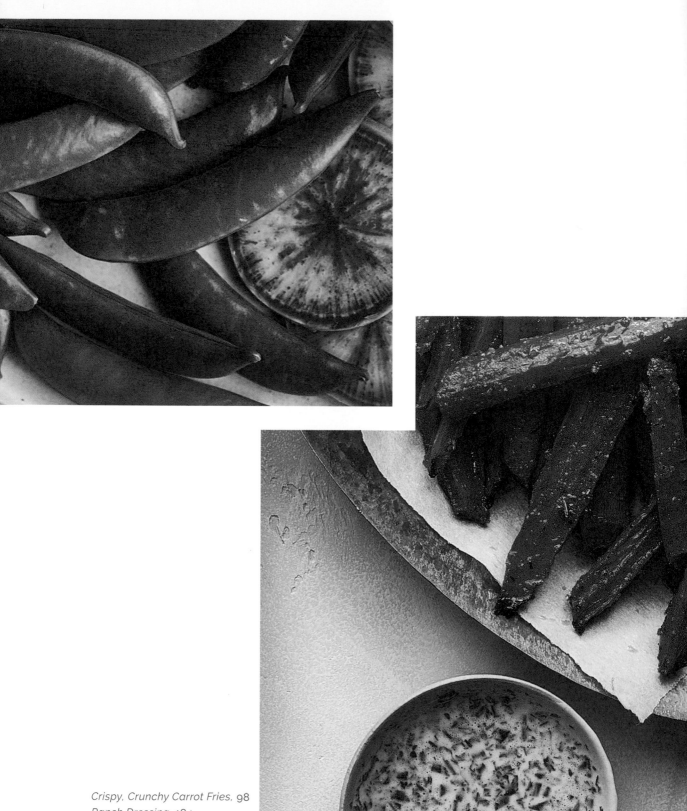

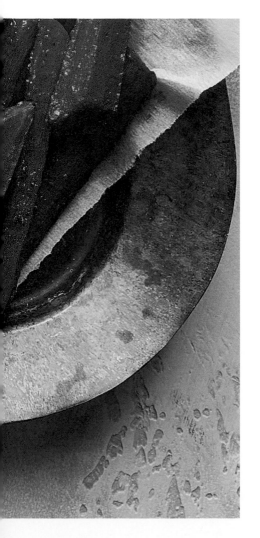

CHAPTER 3

The 21-Day Elimination Diet Meal Plan

The three-week meal plan provided in this chapter is your guide to getting through the elimination phase of the diet with ease, using a variety of the recipes in this book. Each day includes three meals plus a snack option for your eating journey. There's also a weekly shopping list to make your trips to the grocery store quick, efficient, and stress-free.

This meal plan will help things run smoothly for you in a few ways. First, many of the recipes yield more than one serving, which means you'll have leftovers during the week so you don't have to cook every day. Most of these meals can be prepped or completely prepared in advance, and will also freeze well, so you can have a meal ready in a pinch, if needed. There are snack suggestions if you get hungry between meals, but they are optional. Snack or don't as you like.

Finally, the grocery lists provided have everything you need to prepare each week's meals. The first week will include staple pantry items—such as avocado oil, apple cider vinegar, broth, and many spices and seasonings—that will be used to prepare many meals over the course of the three-week elimination diet, as well as the other recipes in the book. You'll stock up on these in week one, so prepare for your biggest food shopping bill that week. In weeks two and three fewer pantry items will be needed; you'll be purchasing mostly the fresh ingredients for the week.

If you don't see a specific amount for something on the shopping list, just buy a bottle/jar/can/bag. These are staples that you'll use again and again. For non-staple items that come in packages—things like walnuts and honey—I'll tell you how much you need for the week and you can buy the closest package size.

Drink Up!

Staying hydrated is very important during this elimination diet. Water helps move toxins out of your body, and proper hydration will put more pep in your step (aka give you energy). The quick way to determine how much water you should drink daily is to take your body weight and divide it in half. That's how many ounces of non-caffeinated beverages you need to keep yourself hydrated. For instance, if you weigh 150 pounds, you should be drinking 75 ounces every day.

Water is the most important beverage you can drink. You can start with a glass of warm water in the morning, then get a large cup, measure the ounces, and that can be your standard drinking cup throughout the day. Some other beverages you can enjoy are herbal teas, spa water (water with lemons, cucumbers, mint, or raspberries), mineral or sparkling water, stocks and broth, and an occasional decaf coffee.

Week One Meal Plan

	Breakfast	Lunch	Dinner	Snacks
Monday	Emerald Green Smoothie (page 66)	Fiesta Black Bean Salad (page 112)	Tandoori Chicken Stew (page 148)	Spiced Walnuts (page 92) with apple
Tuesday	Spinach, Zucchini, and Egg Scramble (page 82, double the recipe)	*Leftover* Fiesta Black Bean Salad	*Leftover* Tandoori Chicken Stew	*Leftover* Spiced Walnuts with banana
Wednesday	*Leftover* Spinach, Zucchini, and Egg Scramble	*Leftover* Fiesta Black Bean Salad	Shrimp and Veggie Stir-Fry (page 130)	*Leftover* Spiced Walnuts with apple
Thursday	*Leftover* Spinach, Zucchini, and Egg Scramble	*Leftover* Shrimp and Veggie Stir-Fry	Turkey and Broccoli Skillet (page 154)	Crispy, Crunchy Carrot Fries (page 98)
Friday	Emerald Green Smoothie	*Leftover* Shrimp and Veggie Stir-Fry	Eggroll Soup (page 158)	*Leftover* Crispy, Crunchy Carrot Fries
Saturday	Sweet and Savory Breakfast Hash (page 78)	*Leftover* Turkey and Broccoli Skillet	*Leftover* Eggroll Soup	*Leftover* Crispy, Crunchy Carrot Fries
Sunday	*Leftover* Sweet and Savory Breakfast Hash	*Leftover* Turkey and Broccoli Skillet	*Leftover* Eggroll Soup	*Leftover* Spiced Walnuts with banana

Week One Shopping List

Canned & Bottled Items

Black beans, 2 (14-ounce) cans

Coconut aminos, 1 (16-ounce) bottle

Coconut milk, full-fat, unsweetened,
2 (14-ounce) cans

Worcestershire sauce, 1 small bottle

Eggs & Dairy Alternatives

Almond milk, plain unsweetened,
½ gallon

Eggs, large, 8

Meat, Poultry & Seafood

Chicken, ground, 1 pound

Chicken, 4 leg quarters

Pork, ground, 1 pound

Shrimp, peeled and
deveined, 1 pound

Turkey cutlets, 1 pound

Pantry Items

Arrowroot powder

Avocado oil

Balsamic vinegar

Broth, chicken or vegetable,
24 ounces

Cayenne pepper

Collagen protein powder,
unflavored

Curry powder

Garam masala

Garlic powder

Ginger, ground

Himalayan or sea salt

Onion powder

Sage, dried

Seasoning blend (of choice)

Sesame oil

Sesame seeds

Thyme, dried

Turmeric, ground

Walnuts, 2 cups (9 ounces)

White pepper

Produce

Apples, 3

Bananas, 2

Avocado, 1

Bell pepper, orange, 1

Bell pepper, yellow, 1

Broccoli crowns, 5

Cabbage, 2 heads

Carrots, about 7

Cilantro, 1 bunch

Dates, pitted, 4

Garlic, 1 head

Ginger, fresh, 1 (2-inch) piece

Kale, 2 bunches

Lemon, 1

Lime, 1

Onion, 1 large

Onion, red, 1 small

Onions, white or yellow, 2 small

Poblano pepper, 1

Spinach, 1 large bag

Sweet potatoes, 2 medium

Tomatoes, cherry, 1 pint

Zucchini, 2 medium

Week Two Meal Plan

	Breakfast	Lunch	Dinner	Snacks
Monday	Spiced Apple, Kale, and Turkey Sauté (page 80)	Curried Lentil Stew (page 108)	Chili-Glazed Salmon with Roasted Veggies (page 140)	Sweet Potato "Toast" with Avocado (page 100)
Tuesday	*Leftover* Spiced Apple, Kale, and Turkey Sauté	*Leftover* Curried Lentil Stew	*Leftover* Chili-Glazed Salmon with Roasted Veggies	*Leftover* Sweet Potato "Toast" with Avocado
Wednesday	*Leftover* Spiced Apple, Kale, and Turkey Sauté	*Leftover* Curried Lentil Stew	Beef and Kale Red Curry (page 170)	*Leftover* Sweet Potato "Toast" with Avocado
Thursday	Red Velvet Smoothie (page 68)	*Leftover* Beef and Kale Red Curry	Nutty Chicken Lettuce Wraps (page 146)	Zucchini Hummus (page 101) with carrots
Friday	Red Velvet Smoothie	*Leftover* Beef and Kale Red Curry	Turkey Veggie Herb Burger Patties with Sweet Potatoes (page 156)	*Leftover* Zucchini Hummus with carrots
Saturday	Bacon, Mushroom, and Egg Mini Quiches (page 83)	*Leftover* Nutty Chicken Lettuce Wraps	*Leftover* Turkey Veggie Herb Burger Patties with Sweet Potatoes	*Leftover* Zucchini Hummus with carrots
Sunday	*Leftover* Bacon, Mushroom, and Egg Mini Quiches	*Leftover* Nutty Chicken Lettuce Wraps	*Leftover* Turkey Veggie Herb Burger Patties with Sweet Potatoes	*Leftover* Zucchini Hummus with carrots

Week Two Shopping List

Canned & Bottled Items

Coconut milk, full-fat, unsweetened, 2 (14-ounce) cans

Fish sauce, 1 (6.75-ounce) jar

Red curry paste, 1 (4-ounce) jar

Rice vinegar, 1 bottle

Tahini, 1 jar

Tomatoes, diced, 2 (14-ounce) cans

Thai chili sauce, 1 jar

Eggs

Eggs, large, 6

Meat, Poultry & Seafood

Bacon, 8 ounces

Beef, ground, 1 pound

Chicken, rotisserie, 1

Salmon, 4 fillets

Turkey, ground, 2½ pounds

Pantry Items

Broth, chicken, beef, or vegetable, 8 ounces

Cashews, 1 cup (6 ounces)

Cinnamon, ground

Cocoa or cacao powder, unsweetened

Ghee

Honey, 12 ounces

Lentils, green, 1 cup (about ½ pound)

Produce

Apple, 1

Avocado, 1

Bananas, 2

Beets, 2 large

Bell peppers, red, 2

Bell pepper, yellow, 1

Carrots, 9 large

Cauliflower, 1 head

Chives, 1 bunch

Cucumber, 1 medium

Garlic, 1 head

Lemon, 1

Lettuce, butter leaf, 1 head

Lime, 1

Kale, 3 bunches

Mushrooms, 1 pound

Onion, red, 1

Onions, yellow, 2

Parsley, 1 bunch

Scallions, 1 bunch

Sweet potatoes, 3 large

Sweet potatoes, 9 small

Zucchini, 2 large

Week Three Meal Plan

	Breakfast	Lunch	Dinner	Snacks
Monday	Coconut Quinoa Porridge (page 69)	Crunchy Tuna Salad (page 128)	Stuffed Portobello Burgers (page 124) with Baked Sweet Potato (page 176)	Sweet and Simple Seedy Granola (page 94)
Tuesday	*Leftover* Coconut Quinoa Porridge	*Leftover* Crunchy Tuna Salad	*Leftover* Stuffed Portobello Burgers with Baked Sweet Potato	*Leftover* Sweet and Simple Seedy Granola
Wednesday	*Leftover* Coconut Quinoa Porridge	*Leftover* Stuffed Portobello Burgers with Baked Sweet Potato	Shrimp Curry (page 132)	*Leftover* Sweet and Simple Seedy Granola
Thursday	Chocolate Cherry Smoothie (page 67)	*Leftover* Shrimp Curry	Baked Chicken Sausage with Apples and Potatoes (page 147)	Edible Brownie Batter (page 103) with apple
Friday	Chocolate Cherry Smoothie	*Leftover* Shrimp Curry	Beef Stir-Fry (page 166)	*Leftover* Edible Brownie Batter with apple
Saturday	Banana-Walnut Almond Flour Muffins (page 72)	*Leftover* Baked Chicken Sausage with Apples and Potatoes	*Leftover* Beef Stir-Fry	*Leftover* Edible Brownie Batter with apple
Sunday	*Leftover* Banana-Walnut Almond Flour Muffins	*Leftover* Baked Chicken Sausage with Apples and Potatoes	*Leftover* Beef Stir-Fry	*Leftover* Edible Brownie Batter with apple

Week Three Shopping List

Canned & Bottled Items

Apple sauce, unsweetened, 4 ounces

Black beans, 1 (14.5-ounce) can

Coconut cream, full-fat, 1 (4-ounce) can

Coconut milk, full-fat, unsweetened, 2 (14.5-ounce) cans

Lemon juice, 1 (8-ounce) bottle

Lime juice, 1 (8-ounce) bottle

Red curry paste, 1 jar

Tomatoes, diced, 1 (14-ounce) can

Tuna, low-sodium, 2 (5-ounce) cans (packed in broth or water)

Eggs & Dairy Alternatives

Eggs, large, 2

Frozen Foods

Cherries, 1 cup

Meat, Poultry & Seafood

Beef round or skirt steak, 1½ pounds

Chicken sausage, 4 large

Shrimp, peeled and deveined, 1 pound

Pantry Items

Almond flour

Baking powder

Baking soda

Basil, dried

Coconut flakes, unsweetened

Monk fruit sweetener or honey

Olive oil

Oregano, dried

Pumpkin seeds

Quinoa

Raisins

Sunflower seeds

Vanilla extract

Walnuts

Produce

Apples, 6

Avocado, 1

Bananas, 4

Bell pepper, green, 1

Bell peppers, red, 2

Blueberries, 1 pint

Broccoli crown, 1

Carrots, 4

Celery, 1 pound

Cilantro, 1 bunch

Garlic, 2 heads

Ginger, fresh, 2 (2-inch) pieces

Lemon, 1

Lime, 1

Mushrooms, 8 ounces

Onions, red, 3

Onion, yellow, 1

Portobello mushrooms, 4

Potatoes, fingerling, 1 pound

Scallions, 1 bunch

Snow peas, 1 cup

Spinach, 1 large bag

Strawberries, 1 pint

Sweet potatoes, 7

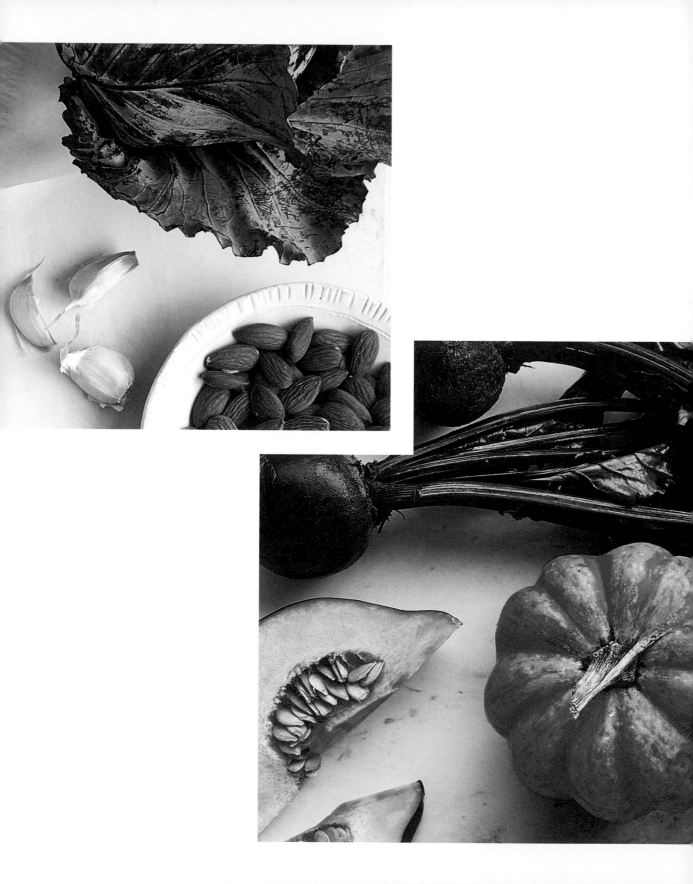

CHAPTER 4

Life After the Elimination Diet

The elimination diet is a short-term diet; it is intended to clear your body of the proteins that are creating an autoimmune response, so you can test them one by one to determine how your body reacts. The reintroduction process is gradual, but it will give you information that would be very difficult to get if you didn't remove the problematic foods first.

hile there are likely some foods that will have to be permanently eliminated from your diet, this journey allows you to understand how profoundly foods affect you. Your body will be communicating with you, sending you signs—but you must pay attention. Listen to how you feel mentally and physically, as these are the ways your body will speak to you. Pay attention to other people's experiences, but remember that what works for one person may not work for another. You are creating your own personalized diet—the one that works specifically for you.

How to Reintroduce

Congratulations on making it through the elimination phase! You can now start the process of customizing your diet. Before moving on, it's a good idea to honestly evaluate how you are feeling. Ask yourself these questions:

- Do I have more energy?

- Am I sleeping better?

- Has there been a change to my gastrointestinal system? Any difference in reflux? Less abdominal bloating? Bowels moving easier?

- Any changes in brain fog?

- Have my food cravings changed?

Taking an inventory of how you feel before introducing eliminated foods back into your diet helps you establish a baseline before reintroduction.

After 21 days of elimination, your immune system should be calmer, your brain should be functioning better, and you may be feeling you generally have more energy. Now it's the exciting time to add foods back. This is a very structured and methodical reintroduction that consists of two parts: first, reintroducing the food; second, evaluating your symptoms. This process takes patience, as moving too quickly can cause confusion about what is causing your symptoms.

I've included a Food Journal template on page 53 to help guide you as you move through the reintroduction process. There is no specific order in which you should reintroduce foods. Start with the food you are missing the most. The important part is to reintroduce foods *one at a time*, and allow at least three days for your body to respond, as it can take this long for the immune system to react.

You will start by having a reasonable serving of the new food on day one. On day two, you will double that serving. For example, if you want to reintroduce yogurt, on day one you will have one 4-ounce to 6-ounce serving of yogurt. On day two you will increase it to two 4-ounce to 6-ounce servings. On day three, you won't have any yogurt, but you will continue to evaluate how you feel throughout the process. (You will not add anything on day three because you want to evaluate how you feel and make sure you are truly symptom-free.)

You should not introduce any new food until you are sure that your first food is not causing any symptoms. So an equally important part of the reintroduction is to document how you feel. If you do have symptoms, remove that food and do not introduce a new food until you return to baseline—however many days that takes for you. If you are certain you do not have symptoms, then you can consider that food acceptable and start with the next food reintroduction.

This means reintroducing each new food will take at least three days. If you experience symptoms, it will take longer, because you must give yourself time to return to baseline before you reintroduce another new food. This is a constant learning process to help you fine-tune your diet, so be patient—it will be worth it.

How to Track Your Symptoms

The key to understanding your symptoms is to write them down. As much as you may think you will remember, writing them down will remove any question or confusion. Documenting as much information as you can makes putting the pieces of a puzzle together easier. The vital pieces of data include:

- The food introduced

- The amount eaten

- The day and time of introduction

- Any symptoms, such as changes in energy (improved or decreased), acid reflux, bloating, abdominal cramping, brain fog, sleeping changes, or constipation

- Any other changes that may play a role in the symptoms you experience, such as medication adjustments, adding a new supplement, not allowing enough time for sleep, or unusual stressors

It is crucial during this phase that if you do have a symptom, you immediately remove the food until your symptoms return to baseline. You can always retest a food at another time.

A common mistake during this time is to write off the connection between food and symptoms, ignoring the way your body is communicating with you. In many cases it may be the foods you eat most frequently or some comfort foods that your body is reacting to. It's common for people to attribute their symptoms to something else, often because they don't want to admit that a food that's important to them is causing symptoms. When you're tracking, be consistent, write it down, and be honest with yourself. Use the Symptom Tracker template on page 57 to track your symptoms.

From Diet to Lifestyle

When you complete the elimination and reintroduction phases, you will have created the diet that works specifically for you. It's your You Diet. Now that you know, you can't un-know the impact food has on the way your body functions. You have developed the template for what foods work well for you and what foods you should avoid moving forward to prevent your symptoms from returning. Just as Hashimoto's is a condition that is lifelong, what you have discovered is not a short-term fix, but a way of eating that you can rely on for a lifetime.

There will certainly be times when you veer from what you have discovered here. There will be times when you eat something that you already know is not going to serve you well. It will happen. When it does, be prepared to feel one or more of your old symptoms return. The timing of your symptoms will depend on a few factors, such as how much of the food you ate, how often you ate it, and what else you had with the food. Remember, it can take as long as three days before you start to experience symptoms, so be ready.

Also understand that if you've veered from your You Diet, all is not lost. You can just pick it up again. Whether it's a meal, a day, or a few weeks that you've gone off your plan, use the information you've gathered as fuel to get you back on track. You can always come back to what you know works best for you.

FOOD JOURNAL

DAY/DATE	TIME	FOOD OR BEVERAGE	SERVING SIZE	MEDICATIONS/ SUPPLEMENTS	COMMENTS/SYMPTOMS
BREAKFAST					
LUNCH					

FOOD JOURNAL (continued)

DAY/DATE	TIME	FOOD OR BEVERAGE	SERVING SIZE	MEDICATIONS/ SUPPLEMENTS	COMMENTS/SYMPTOMS
DINNER					
SNACKS					

Tips for Social Success

Being on an elimination diet doesn't mean you have to be secluded. You can still enjoy time with other people. Social time is an opportunity to enjoy the company of the people around you, rather than focus on what's available to eat.

Dining out. With careful planning, you can make eating out work on an elimination diet, though there are challenges. Before you go to a restaurant, review the menu (most restaurants put their menus online). In most cases you can find a grilled meat or fish and a vegetable that will be appropriate. Once you are seated, ask questions. The servers are there to provide you with a pleasant experience, so ask about what kind of oil they use, if they put butter in their vegetables, or if they have olive oil for a salad dressing. Don't be afraid to ask for substitutions or to just leave certain foods off the plate. They are usually happy to help.

Social gatherings. There are ways to make these manageable without throwing you off your diet. Always eat before you go. If you are not hungry while at a gathering, you can be selective about what foods you eat while there. Ask if you can contribute something, then bring a dish that you know you can eat without getting off-track. Chances are you will not be the only one who will enjoy your contribution.

Cooking for others. Think of this as an opportunity to show others that your foods taste delicious and are also healthy. There is no need to prepare separate meals for yourself, as there are many recipes in this book that can work for everyone.

A Lifelong Journey

It is possible that over time, even if you are following your plan precisely, your symptoms may change. You may start to feel your old, familiar, and terrible symptoms show up again. This is not because you've done something wrong, but because your nutritional needs can change over time. As you age, your hormones change, life stressors change, your body changes, and your diet may need adjusting.

The 21-day elimination diet is a structured process that you can come back to, to reevaluate what is affecting you. You can use it as a reset to get back on track or to reexamine what foods work for you and what foods do not. In fact, it's a good practice to complete the 21-day process once a year to recognize which foods could be contributing to a symptom that's creeping in, before it gets too awful. Additionally, this may be a time to dive deeper, doing a Next-Level Elimination to temporarily remove other foods that could cause an immune reaction, including nuts, seeds, eggs, all grains, nightshades, beans, and legumes.

While an elimination diet is not an easy process, it is a safe way to gain peace of mind about how to feed your body. It allows the body to rest, reset, and refocus. You know it has worked for you before, so you can lean on this diet process at any time to reestablish and reaffirm your You Diet.

We know that diet is a major factor in your progress toward resolving your Hashimoto's symptoms. It takes dedication, planning, and persistence. However, there are many other lifestyle factors that will contribute. Stress, sleep quality, and activity or exercise also play roles in the healing process. After focusing on diet, ease into the other lifestyle factors and work on incorporating them one at a time. You don't have to master everything at once.

SYMPTOM TRACKER

DATE								
ACID REFLUX								
ANXIETY								
BLOATING/GAS								
NASAL CONGESTION								
ABDOMINAL CRAMPING								
HEADACHES								
INCREASED HEART RATE/ PALPITATIONS								
OTHER								

Plan Your Meals

As I've stressed again and again throughout this book, having a plan is extremely important. Just like using your GPS when you're on a road trip, a structured meal plan provides you with clear, precise directions to help you navigate your meals without stress and panic.

The meal plans provided in chapter 3 are your guide to getting through the elimination phase. Going forward, meal planning is one of the keys to success when preparing for a symptom-free life. It is the map that provides direction and takes the guesswork out of what to eat when you are hungry.

Planning your meals every day may seem time-consuming and overwhelming, but it is crucial. As you move through the elimination phase you can lean on the meal plans provided here, and when you start the reintroduction phase you will start to create your own meal plans.

Follow these steps to make your own meal plans.

1. Set aside some time each week, preferably on the day before you're going grocery shopping, to sit down and plan your meals and snacks for the week. It will take some time on the front end, but this is critical to making your weekly meals (and your weekly shopping) go smoothly.
2. Remember to look at your calendar for the upcoming week. Plan to prepare meals on days when you have a little more time, so you will have things in the refrigerator and freezer for the days when you have less time.
3. Next, include leftovers in your meal plans. Sometimes the leftovers will be from what you prepared the day before, sometimes it will mean pulling a previously prepared meal from the freezer.
4. Add only one to three new recipes each week. This keeps you from getting frustrated in the kitchen.
5. Once you have figured out your meals for the week, write down what ingredients you need. Check what you have already in the pantry, refrigerator, and freezer, then make a detailed list of what you need to buy at the supermarket or online.

Remember, a meal plan is a tool to make the cooking simpler. Once you create and learn your process, it will get much easier.

Manage Your Stress

Stress is an inevitable part of life. There are different kinds of stressors: metabolic stressors within the body (such as unbalanced blood sugar) and stressors outside the body. The daily stressors we are most familiar with are the outside, psychological stressors, including the morning rush to get everyone out of the house on time, traffic, work deadlines, sick family members, and other unexpected challenges.

These stressors affect thyroid function in multiple ways. Stress slows down the production of TSH, the hormone produced by the pituitary gland to tell the thyroid to produce T4 hormone. In addition, stress decreases the conversion of T4 to T3. And the stress hormone cortisol, when elevated, causes low-grade inflammation.

On the bright side, research shows that it's not the stressor that causes these problems, but the way you perceive stress. This means that your perception of stress can increase—or decrease—the way your body reacts physiologically. Luckily, there are some beneficial stress-relieving activities that you can do just about anywhere. You can include as many of these as you want every day.

- Deep breathing (breathing in so deep that it moves your abdomen and feels as if you are breathing into your toes)
- Meditation
- Yoga
- Walking in nature
- Playing with pets
- Laughing

Embrace Exercise

Activity and movement are crucial to balancing Hashimoto's symptoms for two main reasons. First, exercise is a way to strengthen the immune system. This immunity boost can decrease inflammation, which is a primary concern when working to decrease autoimmune antibodies from Hashimoto's.

Second, regular activity is an excellent way to balance blood sugar. Since it's common for people with Hashimoto's to have blood sugar dysregulation, exercise is an easy tool that can be used daily to help. Gentle exercising, such as walking, just after eating is an efficient way to decrease blood sugar.

However, this is not a time to jump into an intense exercise routine, even if you have the energy. Remember, when the thyroid is struggling, the adrenal glands also take a hit. High-intensity exercise and overtraining can make your path to healing longer, as your adrenals try to keep up with the physical demands. The best exercises for you currently are the ones that keep you moving, slightly increase your heart rate, and keep you flexible. These include walking, yoga, Pilates, and gentle weight training. If you have been doing other exercises and feel energized afterward, feel free to continue doing these as long as they feel good in your body. However, if you feel worn out afterward you may be overdoing it.

Prioritize Sleep

Sleep is an underrated commodity. Many things happen during sleep, such as detoxification of the brain, healing, growth, and repair of all parts of the body. Yet it is often neglected in our busy lives. If you are not allowing for at least seven to nine hours of sleep each night, it is imperative that you adjust your schedule to make more time for sleep.

If you are having difficulty sleeping, here are a few sleep hygiene tips.

Put down your phone, laptop, tablet, or computer. The light from these devices can interfere with your body's production of melatonin, the sleep hormone. Plan to be off all devices for at least one hour before bedtime.

Make sure your room is dark and cool. The light from alarm clocks, night lights, or other lights in the room can affect your sleep quality. A sleeping mask can be a simple tool to help. In addition, the temperature should be appropriate for you to be comfortable throughout the night.

If you have difficulty staying asleep, there are supplements that can help. Magnesium, melatonin, and lavender can help. In addition, GABA or progesterone can also be useful to increase the quality of your sleep. Talk to your health care provider about getting started with one of these, before considering a sleeping medication.

Detox Your Environment

When it comes to detoxifying, it's important for other aspects of your life, too, not just your food. There are a few easy places to start to clean out the toxins in your environment.

Plastic

Begin in the kitchen by eliminating as much plastic as you can. There are clearly some advantages to using plastic; however, it can be detrimental to your hormones. Replace your plastic food storage containers with glass, your plastic water bottle with stainless steel, and plastic zip-top bags with reusable silicone ones.

Cleaning Supplies

Household cleaning supplies are the next place to clean up. Many of the cleaners we use are made with common allergens and irritants and have been shown to contribute to cancer. Some basic kitchen ingredients, such as baking soda and vinegar, can do a fine job cleaning. If you are looking to buy greener cleaning supplies, visit the Environmental Working Group's website for an up-to-date list of products.

Makeup and Skin Care

Anything you put on your skin, from makeup to lotion to soap, should be evaluated. These products have chemicals that are not regulated and that can lead to hormone disruption. Your skin is your largest organ and is highly absorbent, meaning anything that touches the skin quickly gets absorbed directly into your body. The Environmental Working Group is an excellent resource for these products as well.

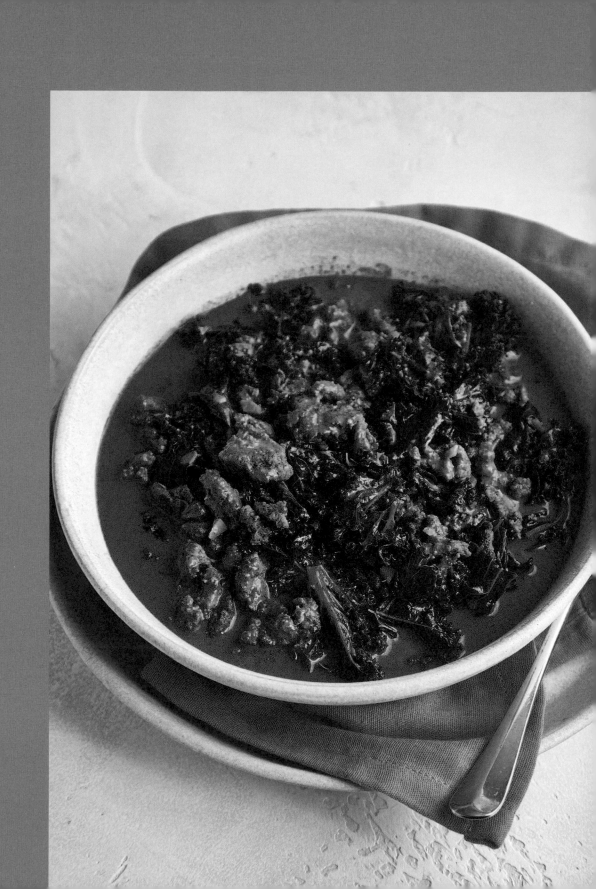

PART TWO

The Recipes

This part of the book is Hashimoto's-friendly recipes that you can use for the elimination diet and beyond. They are all free of dairy, gluten, soy, concentrated sugars, alcohol, and caffeine. The recipes are labeled to identify which meals are quick to prepare, use only one pot, require five or fewer ingredients (excluding salt, pepper, and oil), or are freezer-friendly.

While this elimination diet is not as drastic as some, it is a good place to start so that you can begin to feel better and move forward in building your You Diet. Some recipes are also free of all foods that could trigger the autoimmune process. These recipes will include the "Next-Level Elimination–friendly" label. For others, I've included tips for further eliminating potentially triggering foods (identified by an asterisk), if that's what your body requires. Pepper, cayenne, and jalapeño are always optional. If garlic and onions or their powders cause bloating, you can substitute leeks, green onions, or scallions for onions and eliminate the garlic.

Beef and Kale Red Curry, 170

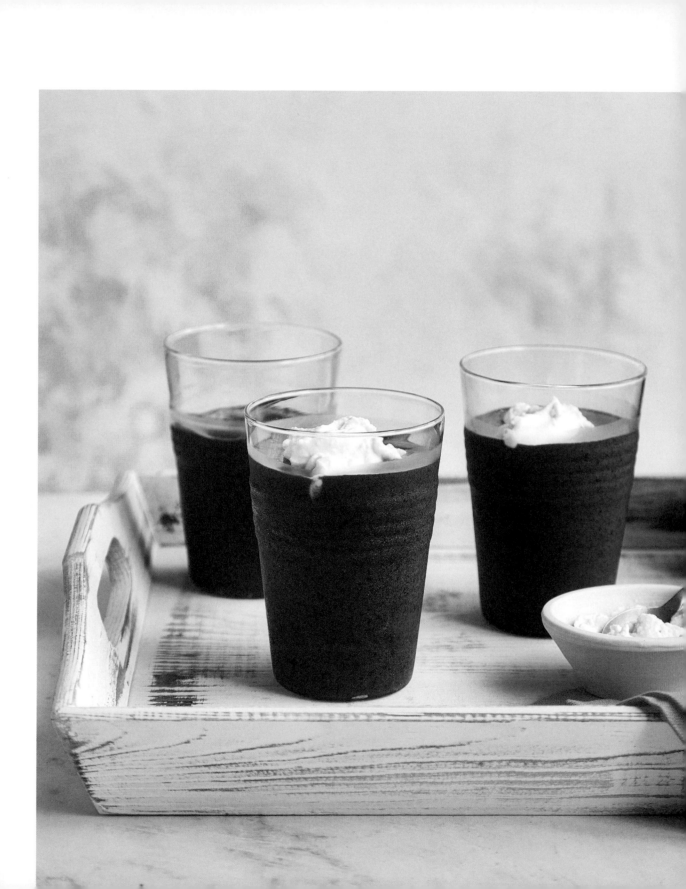

Breakfasts

Emerald Green Smoothie

This smoothie is quick, convenient, and perfect for people who have difficulty eating something in the mornings and can better tolerate a beverage. The spinach and kale make this shake the most beautiful shade of green, while the dates provide a hint of sweetness and the avocado adds a creamy texture that makes it feel like you're drinking an ice cream shake.

¼ cup canned, unsweetened, full-fat coconut milk

¾ cup water

½ cup crushed ice

1 cup spinach

1 cup chopped kale

¼ avocado

2 dates, pitted

1 scoop unflavored collagen protein powder

- ONE POT
- 30 MINUTES OR LESS
- NEXT-LEVEL ELIMINATION–FRIENDLY

Serves 1

Prep time: 7 minutes

Substitution Tip: You can substitute other greens, such as Swiss chard, beet greens, or a mixed green combination. You can also substitute ½ cup frozen spinach in this recipe instead of fresh, to make it even more like ice cream.

Time-Saving Tip: You can buy kale already cut and ready to use in the refrigerated section of the produce aisle.

1. Before measuring, mix the coconut milk well with either a spoon or an immersion blender, to blend the liquid and coconut cream if they are separated.

2. Blend the coconut milk and water in a high-powered blender.

3. Add the ice, spinach, kale, avocado, dates, and protein powder and blend on High until all the ingredients are well blended.

4. Drink right away.

Per serving: Calories: 442; Fat: 19g; Carbohydrates: 26g; Fiber: 6g; Sugar: 11g; Protein: 49g; Sodium: 112mg

Chocolate Cherry Smoothie

This smoothie will make you feel like you are drinking a little piece of heaven, and cheating on breakfast with dessert. The cocoa powder gives it a rich chocolate flavor, the banana provides sweetness, and the cherries add a tart kick to the smoothie.

¼ cup canned, unsweetened, full-fat coconut milk

¾ cup water

½ cup frozen cherries

½ frozen banana

2 tablespoons unsweetened cocoa powder*

1 scoop unflavored collagen protein powder

- ONE POT
- 5 INGREDIENTS OR LESS
- 30 MINUTES OR LESS

Serves 1

Prep time: 7 minutes

1. Before measuring, mix the coconut milk well with either a spoon or immersion blender, to blend the liquid and coconut cream if they are separated.

2. Blend the coconut milk and water in a high-powered blender.

3. Add the cherries, banana, cocoa powder, and protein powder and blend on High until all the ingredients are well blended.

4. Drink right away.

Per serving: Calories: 396; Fat: 14g; Carbohydrates: 30g; Fiber: 6g; Sugar: 14g; Protein: 49g; Sodium: 59mg

Cooking Tip: To freeze your bananas, peel them and place them whole in a zip-top bag. When you are ready to use them, you can easily break them into pieces and throw them in the blender. Frozen bananas can keep in the freezer for up to 3 months.

Next-Level Elimination Tip: Cocoa and cacao are both derived from a bean, which could potentially trigger symptoms. If that's the case, you can substitute carob powder for cocoa to make this recipe Next-Level Elimination–friendly. Carob powder is a cocoa alternative that is made from dried, roasted carob tree pods. You can often find it in health food stores.

Red Velvet Smoothie

If you like red velvet cake, you will love this smoothie. Whether you're using cocoa or carob (the latter making this Next-Level Elimination-friendly), it blends well with beets! The canned coconut milk provides a creamy consistency that resembles ice cream, and the cocoa, banana, and beet combo create a decadent flavor you can only get with this smoothie.

1 large beet

¼ cup canned, unsweetened, full-fat coconut milk

¾ cup water

½ cup crushed ice

1 frozen banana

1 tablespoon unsweetened cocoa powder*

1 scoop unflavored collagen protein powder

- ONE POT
- 5 INGREDIENTS OR LESS
- 30 MINUTES OR LESS

Serves 1

Prep time: 10 minutes

Cook time: 20 minutes

Time-Saving Tip: You can buy beets already peeled and cooked in the produce section of the grocery store. If you'd like to freeze them, dice them and lay the pieces flat on a plate in the freezer until frozen. Then store them in a zip-top bag in the freezer for up to 6 months.

Cooking Tip: For added decadence, top your smoothie with a dollop of coconut whipped cream. Chill 1 can of full-fat coconut milk in the refrigerator overnight. Pour into a mixer or use a hand mixer to whip coconut cream for 3 to 4 minutes until light and fluffy.

1. Preheat the oven to 400°F.

2. Wrap the beet in aluminum foil and bake for 20 minutes. Cool, then cut a slit in the skin, peel it off, and discard. It should easily peel away from the beet. Allow the beet to cool completely before using for the smoothie.

3. Before measuring, mix the coconut milk well with either a spoon or immersion blender, to blend the liquid and coconut cream if they are separated.

4. Blend the coconut milk and water in a high-powered blender. Add the ice, beet, banana, cocoa powder, and protein powder and blend on High until all the ingredients are well blended.

5. Drink right away.

Per serving: Calories: 445; Fat: 13g; Carbohydrates: 41g; Fiber: 7g; Sugar: 23g; Protein: 49g; Sodium: 135mg

Coconut Quinoa Porridge

This recipe is pure comfort food. The combination of coconut milk, vanilla extract, and blueberries provides just the right amount of sweetness, while the salt balances out the flavors. The pumpkin seeds provide a bit of crunch and are also a great source of zinc.

1½ cups quinoa*

4 cups water

1 cup canned, unsweetened, full-fat coconut milk

¼ teaspoon Himalayan or sea salt

¼ teaspoon alcohol-free vanilla extract

1 cup blueberries, fresh or frozen

¼ cup raw pumpkin seeds*

- ONE POT
- 30 MINUTES OR LESS

Serves 6

Prep time: 2 minutes

Cook time: 25 minutes

Time-Saving Tip: Instead of rinsing the quinoa before cooking, place it in a saucepan with water. Add enough water so it covers the quinoa by at least ½ inch and leave it overnight. The next morning, drain the quinoa with a fine colander, then begin the cooking process. This can reduce the cooking time by about 5 minutes.

1. Place the quinoa in a fine colander and rinse for at least 30 seconds to remove the bitter coating naturally found on quinoa.

2. In a 2-quart pot over high heat, pour in the quinoa, water, coconut milk, and salt. Cover and bring to a boil. Reduce the heat to a simmer and cook for 20 minutes more.

3. Stir in the vanilla and blueberries and cook for 3 to 4 minutes more.

4. Stir in the pumpkin seeds and serve warm.

5. This porridge can be kept in an airtight container in the refrigerator for up to 7 days. To reheat, add ¼ cup water per serving and place in a saucepan over low heat on the stove, or microwave in a bowl until warm.

Per serving (1½ cups): Calories: 280; Fat: 14g; Carbohydrates: 33g; Fiber: 4g; Sugar: 3g; Protein: 8g; Sodium: 87mg

Tahini Squash Porridge

This porridge is a great warm breakfast that will make you feel cozy inside. It has warming flavors like ginger, cinnamon, and turmeric that will make you feel like cuddling up by a fire. These ingredients are also calming and healing for the immune system. This recipe is a great one to double for nearly a week's worth of breakfasts.

1½ cups water, divided

2 cups peeled and diced butternut squash

4 tablespoons unsweetened shredded coconut

2 tablespoons chia seeds*

1 teaspoon ground cinnamon

2 teaspoons ground ginger

½ teaspoon ground turmeric

¼ teaspoon Himalayan or sea salt

2 tablespoons tahini*

2 scoops unflavored collagen protein powder

1. Put ½ cup of water in a 2-quart saucepan over high heat, cover, and bring to a boil. Add the butternut squash and lower the heat to medium-low. Cover and cook until the butternut squash is easy to pierce with a fork, 5 to 8 minutes. Drain.

2. While the butternut squash is cooking, combine the shredded coconut, chia seeds, cinnamon, ginger, turmeric, and salt in a blender until you get a flour-like consistency. Add the remaining 1 cup of water to the blender and let the ingredients sit 10 to 12 minutes, until a gel forms.

3. Once the gel has formed, add the cooked squash, tahini, and protein powder to the blender and blend until well combined, creating a porridge.

4. Pour the porridge into your saucepan and heat over medium heat, stirring occasionally, until it starts to bubble, about 5 minutes. Remove from the heat and serve warm.

5. Leftovers can be stored in an airtight container in the refrigerator for up to 7 days. To reheat, add ¼ cup of water per serving and place in a saucepan over low heat on the stove, or microwave in a bowl until warm.

Per serving (1½ cups): Calories: 494; Fat: 21g; Carbohydrates: 31g; Fiber: 12g; Sugar: 4g; Protein: 51g; Sodium: 313mg

· **30 MINUTES OR LESS**

Serves 2

Prep time: 5 minutes, plus 10 minutes to gel

Cook time: 15 minutes

Time-Saving Tip: Buy butternut squash already peeled and diced in the refrigerated produce section.

Next-Level Elimination Tip: Tahini is made by grinding sesame seeds into a fine paste. Because seeds can potentially trigger symptoms, you can replace the tahini with coconut butter or coconut cream. Additionally, chia seeds could be problematic. Use 1 tablespoon of gelatin powder instead to help thicken the porridge and make this recipe Next-Level Elimination–friendly.

Banana-Walnut Almond Flour Muffins

This recipe is a spin on traditional banana bread that uses the natural sweetness of applesauce and bananas, enhanced by vanilla extract and cinnamon. The healthy fats in almond flour, egg yolks, and walnuts aid in stabilizing blood sugar, and the walnuts also provide a satisfying crunch. These muffins are a great on-the-go breakfast option that will keep you feeling full for hours.

1¼ cups almond flour*
2 teaspoons baking powder
½ teaspoon baking soda
1 teaspoon ground cinnamon
½ cup unsweetened applesauce

2 eggs*
½ teaspoon alcohol-free vanilla extract
3 ripe bananas, peeled and mashed
¼ cup chopped walnuts*

1. Preheat the oven to 350°F. Line a 12-cup muffin tin with parchment paper muffin liners.

2. In a medium bowl, stir together the almond flour, baking powder, baking soda, and cinnamon.

3. In a large bowl, with an electric mixer, blend the applesauce, eggs, vanilla, and bananas until just mixed, being careful not to overmix. If you don't have a mixer, stir well with a whisk. Gently fold the dry ingredients and walnuts into the wet ingredients until they are well blended.

4. Using a large spoon, spoon batter into each muffin cup until the batter is evenly divided among the 12 muffins. Bake for 45 minutes, until the tops of the muffins are lightly browned. Enjoy warm.

5. Store in the refrigerator for up to 7 days. Warm them in a toaster oven or microwave when you're ready to eat.

Per serving (2 muffins): Calories: 212; Fat: 12g; Carbohydrates: 21g; Fiber: 4g; Sugar: 10g; Protein: 7g; Sodium: 133mg

Makes 12 muffins

Prep time: 10 minutes

Cook time: 45 minutes

Cooking Tip: Bananas that are ripe have more natural sweetness. For optimum flavor, let your bananas ripen until about half the banana starts to get brown.

Substitution Tip: If you're not a fan of walnuts, you can leave them out completely or substitute any other nut or seed that you enjoy.

Apple-Carrot Breakfast Muffins

These muffins are great to always have on hand because they are packed with nutrients that will make you feel good. They have natural sweetness from coconut, carrots, apples, and raisins, all enhanced by the vanilla extract. They have the perfect crunch and make a delicious breakfast or snack.

½ cup coconut flour

1 teaspoon baking soda

1 teaspoon Himalayan or sea salt

4 tablespoons ground cinnamon

1 cup shredded unsweetened coconut

3 to 4 carrots

2 small apples, cored

8 eggs*

1 teaspoon alcohol-free vanilla extract

½ cup coconut oil, melted

1¼ cups raisins

1. Preheat the oven to 350°F. Line a 12-cup muffin tin with parchment paper muffin liners.

2. In a large bowl, stir together the coconut flour, baking soda, salt, cinnamon, and shredded coconut.

3. Into a medium bowl, grate the carrots and apples. Add the eggs and vanilla and stir until well combined. Add the coconut oil.

4. Stir the wet ingredients into the dry ingredients and mix well. Add the raisins and stir well.

5. Using a large spoon, spoon batter into each muffin cup until the batter is evenly divided among the 12 muffins. Bake for 20 to 25 minutes or until the muffins begin to brown. Remove from the oven and allow to cool completely before handling.

6. These can be stored in an airtight container in the refrigerator for up to 5 days, or frozen for up to 3 months. To reheat, thaw for 30 minutes at room temperature, then toast them in the oven or toaster oven, or warm them in the microwave.

Per serving (2 muffins): Calories: 570; Fat: 39g; Carbohydrates: 51g; Fiber: 14g; Sugar: 27g; Protein: 13 g; Sodium: 649mg

· FREEZER-FRIENDLY

Makes 12 muffins

Prep time: 15 minutes

Cook time: 25 minutes

Cooking Tip: These muffins can be made into a breakfast loaf and baked for 50 to 60 minutes in a loaf pan, or until a toothpick comes out clean.

Substitution Tip: Instead of raisins, you can use dried cranberries. While these often have sugar added to them, they are well balanced with healthy fats and protein in this recipe to prevent blood sugar fluctuations.

Chicken and Avocado Lettuce Burritos

Sage mixed with onion and garlic provides an unmatched savory flavor that makes this the perfect meal for breakfast—or beyond. Butter leaf lettuce is flexible, so it can be easily rolled, and works perfectly as a tortilla substitute because it holds together well. Plantain Tortillas (page 178) would also be good to wrap these breakfast burritos. The filling for this recipe is a great one to double, giving you leftovers to freeze.

1 tablespoon avocado oil

1 pound ground chicken

½ small onion, diced

½ cup shredded carrots

½ cup chopped mushrooms

½ teaspoon dried sage

¼ to ½ teaspoon Himalayan or sea salt

1 garlic clove, minced

8 large leaves butter leaf or Romaine lettuce, washed and separated

3 tablespoons chopped fresh cilantro

1 large avocado, pitted and sliced

1. In a large sauté pan or skillet over medium heat, heat the avocado oil. Add the ground chicken, onion, carrots, mushrooms, sage, salt, and garlic. Sauté for 10 minutes, until the chicken is cooked and the vegetables are tender.

2. Spoon the chicken mixture into the lettuce leaves, then top with cilantro and avocado.

3. Fold the bottom of the leaf up, then roll the sides in like a burrito.

4. Once cooled, store the remaining filling in an airtight container in the refrigerator for up to 5 days or in a zip-top bag for up to 3 months. When ready to eat, thaw in the refrigerator, then warm in a pan on the stove or a bowl in the microwave and wrap up your burrito.

Per serving (2 burritos): Calories: 240; Fat: 12g; Carbohydrates: 7g; Fiber: 4g; Sugar: 2g; Protein: 28g; Sodium: 208mg

- ONE POT
- 30 MINUTES OR LESS
- FREEZER-FRIENDLY
- NEXT-LEVEL ELIMINATION–FRIENDLY

Serves 4

Prep time: 10 minutes

Cook time: 10 minutes

Substitution Tip: You can substitute ground turkey, pork, or beef in this recipe.

Sweet and Savory Breakfast Hash

This recipe is a great foundation for a filling, satisfying, and nutrient-packed breakfast. You can play around with different seasonings, such as cinnamon to enhance the sweetness of the sweet potato and apple, or white pepper if you prefer a little kick of spice. In this recipe, I also call for a seasoning blend. My go-to is Herbamare, but you can use whatever blend you prefer. This recipe is a great one to double, giving you leftovers to freeze.

2 to 3 tablespoons avocado oil, divided

1 pound ground chicken or chicken sausage

½ teaspoon dried sage

1 tablespoon seasoning blend of choice, divided

1 medium sweet potato, diced

1 large apple, cored and diced

6 cups shredded greens, such as spinach, kale, arugula, or Swiss chard

1. In a large sauté pan or skillet over medium-high heat, heat 1 to 1½ tablespoons of the avocado oil. Add the chicken and sauté for 5 to 7 minutes, until the chicken has browned. Sprinkle in sage and ½ tablespoon of the seasoning blend. Add the remaining 1 to 1½ tablespoons of avocado oil, then add the sweet potatoes and apple. Cook about 2 minutes, uncovered, stirring to brown.

2. Cover the skillet and lower the heat to medium-low. Cook for 5 to 8 minutes more, stirring once midway, until the sweet potatoes and apples are soft.

3. Uncover and add the greens. Sprinkle with the remaining ½ tablespoon of seasoning blend, cover, and cook for 3 minutes. Uncover and continue to cook for 1 minute more, or until most of the liquid has cooked out. Serve warm.

4. Once cooled, store any remaining hash in an airtight container in the refrigerator for up to 5 days or in a zip-top bag for up to 3 months. When ready to eat, thaw in the refrigerator, then warm in a pan on the stove or a bowl in the microwave oven.

Per serving (1½ cups): Calories: 221; Fat: 9g; Carbohydrates: 9g; Fiber: 2g; Sugar: 2g; Protein: 27g; Sodium: 97mg

- ONE POT
- 30 MINUTES OR LESS
- FREEZER-FRIENDLY
- NEXT-LEVEL ELIMINATION–FRIENDLY

Serves 4

Prep time: 10 minutes

Cook time: 20 minutes

Time-Saving Tip: You can buy sweet potatoes already peeled and diced in the refrigerated produce section.

Substitution Tip: Instead of sweet potatoes, you can use butternut squash, which you can also find peeled and diced.

Spiced Apple, Kale, and Turkey Sauté

This meal blends sweet and savory flavors to satisfy any palate. It is an easy one to make, can be served for breakfast or any other time of the day, and is sure to appease everyone's taste buds. This recipe is a great one to double, giving you leftovers to freeze.

2 tablespoons avocado oil

1 pound ground turkey

1 bunch kale

2 teaspoons ground cinnamon

1 teaspoon ground ginger

½ teaspoon Himalayan or sea salt

¼ teaspoon white pepper* (optional)

1 large apple, cored and diced

1. In a large sauté pan or skillet over medium heat, heat the avocado oil. Add the ground turkey and cook for 10 minutes, breaking apart the meat and stirring throughout.

2. While the meat is cooking, cut the kale by placing 3 leaves on top of one another. Fold in half and cut the spine out of the kale and discard. Then cut the leaves into strips.

3. Add the kale, cinnamon, ginger, salt, and pepper (if using) to the pan, and continue cooking until the meat is no longer pink and the kale is softened, 8 to 10 minutes.

4. Add the apple, then cover and cook for 5 minutes more, until the apple is cooked and soft. Serve warm.

5. Once cooled, store any remaining turkey sauté in an airtight container in the refrigerator for up to 5 days or in a zip-top bag for up to 3 months. When ready to eat, thaw in the refrigerator, then warm in a pan on the stove or a bowl in the microwave.

Per serving (1½ cups): Calories: 253; Fat: 9g; Carbohydrates: 16g; Fiber: 3g; Sugar: 6g; Protein: 29g; Sodium: 321mg

- ONE POT
- FREEZER-FRIENDLY
- NEXT-LEVEL ELIMINATION–FRIENDLY

Serves 4

Prep time: 10 minutes

Cook time: 25 minutes

Substitution Tip: The ground turkey in this recipe can be replaced with ground chicken or ground pork.

Spinach, Zucchini, and Egg Scramble

This recipe is a quick and easy dish for breakfast on a weekday or weekend. Spinach is loaded with vitamin A, and pastured eggs are one of the few food sources of vitamin D. Use seasonal veggies to keep this recipe fresh.

4 teaspoons avocado oil, divided

1 medium zucchini, diced

2 cups fresh spinach or 10 ounces frozen spinach

4 large eggs*

¼ teaspoon Himalayan or sea salt

Pinch black pepper* (optional)

- ONE PAN
- 5 INGREDIENTS OR LESS
- 30 MINUTES OR LESS

Serves 2

Prep time: 5 minutes

Cook time: 10 minutes

Substitution Tip: Other vegetables that could be used in this recipe include yellow squash, grape or diced tomatoes, kale, or Swiss chard. If you can tolerate them, onions or leeks can be added to enhance the flavor.

Next-Level Elimination Tip: If you're eliminating eggs, you can substitute 1 cup of diced chicken, making this recipe Next-Level Elimination–friendly. If you're using raw chicken, cook for 10 minutes or until it's thoroughly cooked. If you're adding cooked chicken, cook until warmed and mixed into the vegetables.

1. In a 10-inch sauté pan or skillet, heat 2 teaspoons of oil over medium heat. Add the zucchini and spinach and sauté for 3 minutes. The water in the zucchini will help cook the spinach.

2. While the veggies are cooking, crack the eggs into a medium bowl, add the salt and pepper (is using), and whisk until well combined.

3. Push the veggies to the side of the pan. Add the remaining 2 teaspoons of oil to prevent the eggs from sticking, then pour the eggs into the pan. Scramble the eggs in the pan, incorporating them into the veggies. Cook, stirring for 2 minutes, then remove from the heat and serve.

4. Once cooled, store the remaining scramble in an airtight container in the refrigerator for up to 5 days. Warm in the microwave.

Per serving (1½ cups): Calories: 271; Fat: 20g; Carbohydrates: 9g; Fiber: 4g; Sugar: 3g; Protein: 18g; Sodium: 496mg

Bacon, Mushroom, and Egg Mini Quiches

This recipe is great to prepare on the weekend in a big batch for a quick grab-and-go weekday breakfast. Mushrooms are one of the few food sources of vitamin D, which helps with the development of thyroid hormones.

1 cup chopped bacon*

1½ cups chopped mushrooms

2 tablespoons chopped scallions

½ teaspoon dried thyme

6 eggs*

½ teaspoon Himalayan or sea salt

Freshly ground black pepper* (optional)

• **30 MINUTES OR LESS**

Makes 12 quiches

Prep time: 5 minutes

Cook time: 20 minutes

Substitution Tip: If you are not a fan of mushrooms, substitute sun-dried tomatoes or finely diced sweet potatoes.

Time-Saving Tip: You can buy bacon already chopped and cooked, which speeds up step 2 in this recipe.

1. Preheat the oven to 350°F. Line a 12-cup muffin tin with parchment paper muffin liners.

2. In a large sauté pan or skillet over medium heat, cook the bacon, mushrooms, scallions, and thyme for 5 to 10 minutes.

3. While the bacon and vegetables are cooking, crack the eggs into a medium bowl, and add the salt and pepper (if using). Whisk until well combined.

4. Spoon the bacon mixture into each muffin cup. Pour the eggs evenly into each muffin cup. Bake for 10 minutes, or until the egg is firm to the touch. Serve warm.

5. Once cooled, store in an airtight container in the refrigerator for up to 5 days. Warm in a toaster oven or microwave.

Per serving (2 quiches): Calories: 205; Fat: 15g; Carbohydrates: 2g; Fiber: 0g; Sugar: 1g; Protein: 16g; Sodium: 804mg

Cheesy Beef and Veggie Breakfast Frittata

This recipe looks fancy, but it's quick and easy. Usually found in health food stores (and easy to get online), nutritional yeast is a flake or powder that brings a cheesy, nutty flavor to everything it's added to. It is the perfect pairing for zucchini and tomatoes. Light yet filling, this frittata makes a great breakfast-for-dinner meal when you're craving breakfast at any time of day.

1 tablespoon avocado oil

½ onion, diced

½ bell pepper*, seeded and diced

½ pound ground beef

1 teaspoon Himalayan or sea salt

1 teaspoon black pepper* (optional)

8 eggs*

3 tablespoons nutritional yeast

1 small zucchini, cubed

1 small Roma tomato*, diced

1. Preheat the oven to 350°F.

2. In an ovenproof sauté pan or skillet, heat the avocado oil over medium-high heat. Add the onions and bell pepper and sauté for about 5 minutes, until soft and fragrant. Add the ground beef and season with salt and black pepper (if using). Cook thoroughly, 5 to 8 minutes.

3. While the meat is cooking, beat the eggs in a large mixing bowl and set aside.

4. Remove the meat and vegetables from the skillet and drain any excess oil.

5. Mix the nutritional yeast, zucchini, tomato, and ground beef mixture into the beaten eggs and stir to mix well.

6. Pour the mixture back into the skillet, place in the oven, and bake for 20 minutes or until the frittata is set and solid in the middle. Remove and serve warm.

7. This can be stored covered in the refrigerator for up to 5 days. Reheat in a toaster oven or microwave.

Per serving (¼ frittata): Calories: 304; Fat: 17g; Carbohydrates: 11g; Fiber: 4g; Sugar: 4g; Protein: 29g; Sodium: 644mg

Serves 4

Prep time: 10 minutes

Cook time: 30 minutes

Substitution Tip: There is really no vegetable that you can't use for this frittata—it's a great catch-all for any vegetables you have in the refrigerator that need to get eaten. A few that I've used are broccoli, cauliflower, mushrooms, leeks, garlic, carrots, spinach, and kale.

Time-Saving Tip: Sautéing the ground beef before making the frittata can save a lot of time. Often, I will sauté the onions, bell peppers, and beef when I am making another meal and store them in the refrigerator until needed. When you're ready to prepare the frittata, it's as quick as mixing up the eggs and other ingredients to bake.

Zucchini Fritters

Zucchini fritters are an easy way to add vegetables to breakfast. Paired with a piece of fruit, they are a great grab-and-go meal and can be eaten warmed or straight from the refrigerator. It's best to start the prep the night before to make it smooth sailing for preparation.

2 medium zucchini

1 tablespoon Himalayan or sea salt

2 eggs*

½ teaspoon dried thyme

1 tablespoon avocado oil

- **5 INGREDIENTS OR LESS**

Serves 2

Prep time: 10 minutes, plus 1 hour to sit

Cook time: 10 minutes

1. Shred the zucchini using a food processor or box grater. Place the shredded zucchini on a clean kitchen towel or napkins and sprinkle with salt. Let sit for at least 1 hour so the salt can pull the water out of the zucchini.

2. Squeeze as much water as possible out of the zucchini and place the zucchini in a medium mixing bowl. Add the eggs and thyme and stir well.

3. In a sauté pan or skillet, heat the oil over medium heat. Form the zucchini mixture into 6 palm-size patties and place them in the skillet. Leave them to cook undisturbed until the bottoms start to turn golden brown, 3 to 5 minutes. Flip and cook on the other side, about 3 minutes. Remove the fritters from the pan when both sides are golden brown. Serve warm.

4. Once cooled, store in an airtight container in the refrigerator for up to 5 days. Reheat in a toaster oven or microwave.

Time-Saving Tip: Shred the zucchini and sprinkle with salt the night before. This allows most of the water to be removed, making it easier to squeeze out the water and prepare the fritters quickly in the morning.

Substitution Tip: You can change the flavor with different seasoning blends. Rather than thyme, ½ teaspoon of taco seasoning or an Italian herb blend gives the fritters an international flair.

Per serving (3 patties): Calories: 219; Fat: 19g; Carbohydrates: 7g; Fiber: 2g; Sugar: 4g; Protein: 8g; Sodium: 315mg

Six-Spice Sausage Patties

This breakfast sausage has a distinct savory flavor that is very satisfying. By making this simple recipe at home, you'll ensure that you get only quality ingredients. Pair these patties with a piece of fruit and handful of walnuts for a portable and convenient breakfast.

1 pound ground pork

1 teaspoon Himalayan or sea salt

1 teaspoon dried sage

1 teaspoon dried basil

1 teaspoon white pepper* (optional)

1 teaspoon garlic powder

1 teaspoon onion powder

½ cup water

1 tablespoon avocado oil

- **30 MINUTES OR LESS**
- **FREEZER-FRIENDLY**
- **NEXT-LEVEL ELIMINATION–FRIENDLY**

Serves 4

Prep time: 10 minutes

Cook time: 10 minutes

Cooking Tip: Rather than making the meat mixture into patties, mix and scramble it with eggs, sweet potatoes, or butternut squash.

1. In a large mixing bowl, put in the pork, salt, sage, basil, pepper (if using), garlic powder, onion powder, and water. Wet your hands and mix all the ingredients together. Form the pork mixture into 8 palm-size patties.

2. In a sauté pan or skillet, heat the oil over medium heat. Fry the patties on one side for 3 to 5 minutes, then flip and fry them on the other side until cooked through, about 3 minutes.

3. Remove from the skillet and serve warm.

4. This is a great recipe to double and freeze. Once cooked, lay the patties on a plate or baking sheet and put it in the freezer. Once frozen, place patties into a zip-top bag for up to 3 months until ready to reheat. Warm in a toaster oven, skillet, or microwave on high heat.

Per serving (2 patties): Calories: 266; Fat: 20g; Carbohydrates: 1g; Fiber: 0g; Sugar: 0g; Protein: 20g; Sodium: 549mg

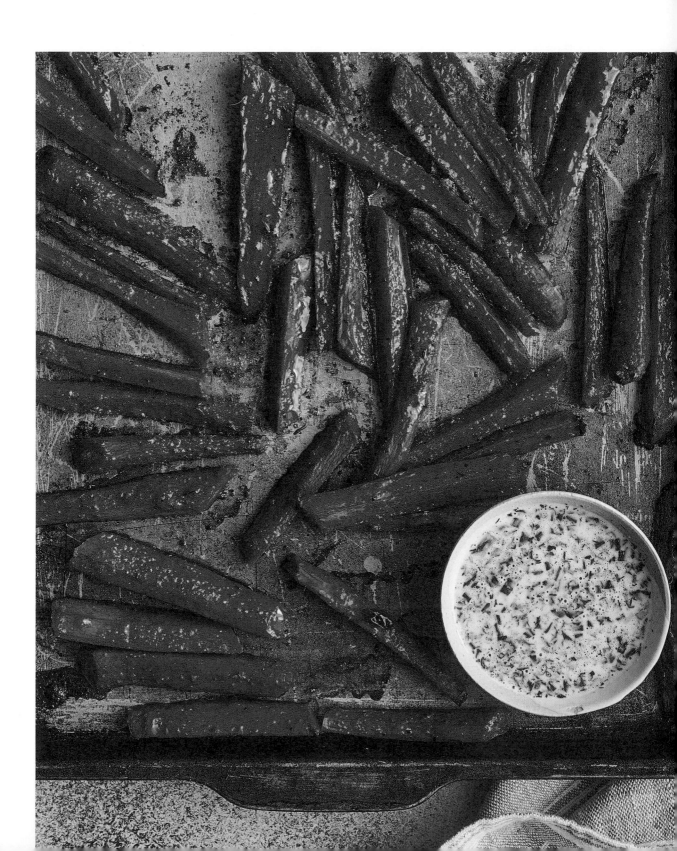

CHAPTER 6
Snacks

Ranch Dressing, 184

Brazil Nut Date Energy Bites

While a bit sweeter than the other recipes in this book, these energy balls get their sweetness naturally from dates, and the carbohydrates are balanced by the healthy fats and protein from the nuts. Brazil nuts provide nature's most abundant source of selenium, which is helpful for thyroid hormone conversion.

1 cup raw Brazil nuts*

1 cup Medjool dates, pitted

½ cup almond butter*

½ teaspoon Himalayan or sea salt

3 tablespoons water, plus more as needed

1. Place the Brazil nuts in a bowl and pour warm water over them to soak for at least 30 minutes to soften for pureeing. Then drain the water.

2. Combine the softened Brazil nuts, dates, almond butter, salt, and 3 tablespoons of water in a food processor and puree until the mixture starts to stick together. You may need to add more water to help the mixture come together.

3. Remove the mixture from the food processor and place it on a cutting board. Using your hands, work to squeeze it all together into one big clump. Break off pieces and roll them into balls about the size of a golf ball. Place the balls on a plate or baking sheet.

4. Refrigerate for about 20 minutes, until they are set. Keep in the refrigerator until you're ready to eat. The balls must stay refrigerated to maintain their consistency.

5. You can double the batch and keep these balls on hand for a quick grab-and-go snack. Store in an airtight container in the refrigerator for up to 1 month.

Per serving (3 balls): Calories: 346; Fat: 25g; Carbohydrates: 31g; Fiber: 5g; Sugar: 22g; Protein: 8g; Sodium: 206mg

· **5 INGREDIENTS OR LESS**

Makes 18 balls

Prep time: 15 minutes, plus 30 minutes to soak and 20 minutes to chill

Substitution Tip: You can substitute any nut or nut butter here to make a similar energy ball.

Cooking Tip: Because of their size, Brazil nuts will take a little more time to process. Be patient with them in the food processor, because you will get the best results if the nuts are processed until creamy.

Spiced Walnuts

These spiced walnuts are a welcome, savory way to enjoy a great plant-based source of omega-3 fatty acids. The savory, umami flavor enhances the meatiness of the nuts, and the cayenne pepper provides a little kick. As always, adjust the spice level to your taste. If the cayenne is too spicy, you can substitute black or white pepper, or just leave out the pepper entirely.

½ teaspoon Himalayan or sea salt

¼ teaspoon cayenne pepper*

½ teaspoon garlic powder

½ teaspoon onion powder

1 tablespoon Worcestershire sauce*

1 tablespoon avocado oil

2 cups walnut halves*

1. Preheat the oven to 325°F and line a baking sheet with parchment paper.

2. In a small bowl, mix the salt, cayenne pepper, garlic powder, and onion powder. Add the Worcestershire sauce and avocado oil to the mixture and stir well.

3. Place the walnuts in a medium bowl. Pour the seasoning blend over them, mixing well to make sure all the walnuts are well coated.

4. Spread the walnuts on the baking sheet in a single layer. Bake for 8 minutes, then stir the walnuts on the baking dish and bake for 5 to 8 minutes more. The walnuts will still look wet; however, as they cool they will absorb the flavoring. Use caution to not overcook, as they will taste burnt.

5. These nuts can be stored in an airtight container in the refrigerator for up to 1 month.

Per serving (⅓ cup): Calories: 159; Fat: 16g; Carbohydrates: 4g; Fiber: 1g; Sugar: 1g; Protein: 3g; Sodium: 184mg

· **30 MINUTES OR LESS**

Makes 2 cups
Prep time: 5 minutes
Cook time: 15 minutes

Substitution Tip: You can substitute pecans for walnuts in this recipe, if you prefer them.

Cooking Tip: Walnuts have plenty of natural oils and will not stick to the baking sheet. But using parchment paper helps them cook more evenly, making them less likely to burn.

Sweet and Simple Seedy Granola

If seeds are not a problem for you, this granola is a great snack, full of healthy fats with a hint of sweetness to satisfy a sweet tooth or craving. Although there is honey and dried fruit in this recipe, the healthy fats and protein from the seeds will keep your blood sugar levels balanced. Pumpkin seeds are also a great source of zinc, to support thyroid hormone conversion from T4 to T3. Feel free to substitute chopped Brazil nuts for the sunflower seeds, for the bonus of selenium.

½ cup raw pumpkin seeds*

½ cup raw sunflower seeds*

½ cup unsweetened coconut flakes

¼ cup honey, warmed

Pinch Himalayan or sea salt

1 teaspoon alcohol-free vanilla extract

1 teaspoon ground cinnamon

½ cup raisins

1. Preheat the oven to 350°F and line a baking sheet with parchment paper.

2. In a medium bowl, mix the pumpkin seeds, sunflower seeds, coconut flakes, warm honey, salt, vanilla, and cinnamon, and stir until everything is well coated.

3. Spread evenly on the baking sheet and cook for 10 to 15 minutes, stirring every 5 minutes. The seeds should be light brown. Use caution to not overcook them, as they will taste burnt.

4. Remove the baking sheet from the oven and stir in the raisins. Continue to stir every few minutes until the granola cools.

5. This granola can be stored in an airtight container for up to 1 month.

Per serving (⅓ cup): Calories: 477; Fat: 30g; Carbohydrates: 42g; Fiber: 7g; Sugar: 30g; Protein: 13g; Sodium: 68mg

• 30 MINUTES OR LESS

Makes 2 cups

Prep time: 5 minutes

Cook time: 15 minutes

Substitution Tip: You can use maple syrup instead of honey to make it vegan. After the granola cools, you can add ¼ cup of cacao nibs for a subtle chocolaty flavor and an added boost of antioxidants.

Time-Saving Tip: Raw nuts may be difficult to find in your supermarket, but they are usually available at health food stores or online. Store them in the refrigerator or freezer until you need them.

Avocado Deviled Eggs

Deviled eggs are an easy snack or appetizer for many occasions. This recipe is a spin on traditional deviled eggs, replacing the mayonnaise with avocado for a healthier fat. You can hard-boil eggs in a batch on the weekend and keep them in the refrigerator all week for snacks and recipes like these, or save yourself some time and buy hard-boiled eggs at the supermarket. Either way, keep in mind that these deviled eggs are best eaten the same day you make them.

1 tablespoon vinegar, any kind

6 eggs*

1 avocado, pitted and cubed

Juice of 1 lime or 2 tablespoons lime juice

2 tablespoons finely chopped red onion

1 teaspoon garlic powder

½ teaspoon Himalayan or sea salt

¼ teaspoon black pepper* (optional)

1. In a 2-quart saucepan over high heat, bring 4 cups of water to a boil. Add the vinegar. Gently place the eggs in the water and boil for 12 minutes. Remove and allow to cool.

2. Peel the cool hard-boiled eggs. Cut them in half lengthwise and scoop the yolks into a medium mixing bowl. Place the egg white halves on a plate.

3. To the egg yolks, add the avocado, lime juice, red onion, garlic powder, salt, and pepper (if using). Use a fork or potato masher to mash all the ingredients together until creamy.

4. With a teaspoon, scoop the avocado mixture into the egg white halves. Alternatively, you can spoon the mixture into a piping bag, or use a zip-top bag and cut the tip off the bottom corner to squeeze the mixture into the eggs.

5. For best flavor, chill in the refrigerator for 20 minutes, then serve.

Per serving (4 egg halves): Calories: 233; Fat: 18g; Carbohydrates: 8g; Fiber: 4g; Sugar: 2g; Protein: 13g; Sodium: 441mg

Serves 3

Prep time: 10 minutes, plus 20 minutes to chill

Cook time: 15 minutes

Time-Saving Tip: Identifying the ripeness of an avocado can be tricky. To make it easier, most grocery stores sell avocado in individual serving containers. Use 3 to 4 of these containers in place of the whole avocado, so you don't have to worry about how ripe your avocado is. You can also purchase peeled hard-boiled eggs, saving you even more time.

Substitution Tip: The lime juice adds a tart citrus kick and also keeps the avocado from browning. Lemon juice works just as well, if you prefer.

Crispy, Crunchy Carrot Fries

These carrot fries are a great way to snack on more veggies throughout the day. They are also a healthy substitute for a side of fries with a burger—and a tastier one, too, since they combine the natural sweetness of carrots with salty and savory spices. Pair them with Ranch Dressing (page 184) for a satisfying snack.

1 pound carrots (about 5 carrots)

2 tablespoons avocado oil

2 tablespoons arrowroot powder

1 teaspoon Himalayan or sea salt

½ teaspoon white pepper* (optional)

½ teaspoon garlic powder

½ teaspoon onion powder

½ teaspoon dried thyme

1. Preheat the oven to 450°F and line a baking sheet with parchment paper.

2. Wash and peel the carrots, then cut them into even sticks, roughly 4 inches long and ½ inch thick.

3. Put the carrot sticks in a large bowl, drizzle with oil, then sprinkle with the arrowroot powder, salt, pepper (if using), garlic powder, onion powder, and thyme. Mix until the carrot sticks are well coated.

4. Spread the carrot sticks in an even layer on the baking sheet. Bake for 15 minutes, then stir the carrots and bake for 5 to 10 minutes more to ensure even cooking. They are done when you can pierce the carrots easily with a fork and they are slightly browned. Remove from the oven and cool for a few minutes. Serve warm.

5. Store in an airtight container in the refrigerator for up to 7 days. Reheat by putting them in the oven or toaster oven at 275°F for 10 minutes or until warm.

Per serving (¼ of recipe): Calories: 128; Fat: 7g; Carbohydrates: 16g; Fiber: 3g; Sugar: 6g; Protein: 1g; Sodium: 546mg

· NEXT-LEVEL ELIMINATION–FRIENDLY

Serves 4

Prep time: 10 minutes

Cook time: 25 minutes

Substitution Tip: For a different flavor, you can substitute parsnips for carrots in this recipe, or use some of each.

Sweet Potato "Toast" with Avocado

There's no need to miss toast when you can make crispy sweet potato toast in the toaster or toaster oven, just the way you would with a slice of bread. This snack is a quick, easy, and versatile option. Enjoy it in the morning with an egg on top for added protein, or for a midday complex carb and healthy fat pick-me-up.

1 medium sweet potato

Pinch Himalayan
    or sea salt

½ avocado, mashed

1 teaspoon
    minced chives

- ONE POT
- 5 INGREDIENTS OR LESS
- 30 MINUTES OR LESS
- NEXT-LEVEL
  ELIMINATION–FRIENDLY

Serves 2

Prep time: 5 minutes

Cook time: 10 minutes

1. Scrub the outside of the sweet potato, dry it, and slice lengthwise into ¼-inch-thick slices.

2. Place in a toaster oven or toaster, on high setting, until lightly browned on both sides. This may take several rounds in the toaster.

3. When browned, sprinkle with salt and spread with avocado. Top with chives and enjoy.

4. Store plain sweet potato slices in the refrigerator in an airtight container for up to 7 days. Reheat by toasting in a toaster oven, toaster, or oven. Top with avocado, chives, and salt before eating.

Per serving (2 slices): Calories: 173; Fat: 11g; Carbohydrates: 18g; Fiber: 6g; Sugar: 3g; Protein: 2g; Sodium: 156mg

Substitution Tip: Once your sweet potato toast is cooked, there are many flavor combos you can top it with instead of avocado. Some of my favorites include sunflower seed butter and bananas, hummus and cherry tomatoes, or Olive-Garlic Tapenade (page 186).

Time-Saving Tip: After your sweet potatoes are sliced, place them in the microwave oven for 30 seconds to get the cooking process started. This will make the toasting go much faster.

Zucchini Hummus

While traditional hummus is made using chickpeas, the zucchini replacement in this recipe is hands down one of the best versions of hummus you will enjoy. Don't be surprised if you find that your vegetable-to-hummus ratio is off, and you're spooning rather than dipping them. And if you do find yourself using a spoon instead of vegetables to scoop, that's okay, too.

2 large zucchini

1 tablespoon avocado oil

1 teaspoon Himalayan or sea salt

½ teaspoon black pepper* (optional)

⅓ cup tahini*

4 garlic cloves

2 tablespoons lemon juice

· 5 INGREDIENTS OR LESS

Serves 4

Prep time: 10 minutes, plus 10 minutes to cool and time to chill

Cook time: 20 minutes

Time-Saving Tip: To speed the process, roast the zucchini one day when you have the oven on for something else, and keep it in the refrigerator for up to 5 days until you are ready to make this hummus.

Cooking Tip: To quickly peel garlic, break the head into individual cloves and put it in a mason jar. Secure the lid and shake vigorously for 15 to 30 seconds. The skins will easily peel right off the cloves.

1. Preheat the oven to 400°F. Line a baking sheet with parchment paper.

2. Cut the zucchini into 2-inch chunks and place them on the baking sheet. Drizzle with avocado oil and sprinkle with salt and pepper (if using). Bake for 20 minutes, then let cool for 10 minutes.

3. Place the roasted zucchini, tahini, garlic, and lemon juice in a food processor or high-powered blender and process until completely smooth.

4. Chill for a couple of hours for best flavor, then serve with veggies.

5. Store in the refrigerator in an airtight container for up to 7 days.

Per serving (½ cup): Calories: 364; Fat: 29g; Carbohydrates: 22g; Fiber: 8g; Sugar: 6g; Protein: 11g; Sodium: 1018mg

Sweet Fried Plantains

Fried plantains are a traditional treat in the Caribbean. Once you taste them, they are likely to become a staple in your house, too. Their natural sugars quickly caramelize and brown, making them crispy on the edges, and the hint of sweetness from the unrefined coconut oil enhances the flavor of the plantains.

1 yellow plantain, ripe

2 tablespoons unrefined coconut oil

¼ teaspoon ground cinnamon

1 tablespoon coconut cream

- **5 INGREDIENTS OR LESS**
- **30 MINUTES OR LESS**
- **NEXT-LEVEL ELIMINATION–FRIENDLY**

Serves 2

Prep time: 5 minutes, plus time to cool

Cook time: 6 minutes

1. Line a plate with a paper towel and set it to the side. Peel and slice the plantain into ½-inch slices.

2. In a sauté pan or skillet, heat the coconut oil over medium-high heat. Place the plantains in the skillet and fry them for 2 to 3 minutes on each side, being careful not to burn them. Place the plantains on the paper-towel-lined plate to cool, then transfer them to a serving bowl.

3. Sprinkle the plantains with cinnamon and drizzle the coconut cream on top. Serve warm.

Per serving (½ plantain): Calories: 265; Fat: 16g; Carbohydrates: 34g; Fiber: 2g; Sugar: 18g; Protein: 1g; Sodium: 6mg

Substitution Tip: Plantains pair well with a sweet or savory flavor. Instead of adding cinnamon and coconut cream, you can add a pinch each of onion powder, garlic powder, and Himalayan or sea salt for a savory flavor.

Cooking Tip: Although plantains look like bananas, they are considered ripe when the skins are mostly black with just a little yellow.

Edible Brownie Batter

When you just need something decadent, this recipe is it. Strawberries are an excellent source of vitamin C, which is necessary for thyroid hormone production, and the black beans add a significant amount of fiber to this sweet treat. Additionally, monk fruit—a natural sweetener made from lo han fruit—will sweeten the batter without raising blood sugar.

¾ cup monk fruit sweetener*

⅓ cup water

Pinch Himalayan or sea salt

1 (14-ounce) can black beans*, rinsed and drained

⅓ cup unsweetened cocoa powder*

¼ cup coconut cream

1 teaspoon alcohol-free vanilla extract

1 cup strawberries

• **30 MINUTES OR LESS**

Serves 3

Prep time: 7 minutes

Cook time: 5 minutes

Substitution Tip: If you'd rather use a different fruit, this batter works as a great dip for apples and bananas, too.

Cooking Tip: If you are unable to find granulated monk fruit sweetener at your grocery store or health food store, honey or maple syrup make good substitutes. If you're using either of these, you can eliminate step 1, as they do not need to be dissolved in water.

1. In a saucepan, cook the monk fruit sweetener, water, and salt on low heat until the sweetener is completely dissolved, about 5 minutes.

2. In a blender, put in the black beans, monk fruit and water mixture, cocoa powder, coconut cream, and vanilla. Process until smooth. You may need to add water to blend well; add ¼ cup at a time until you're able to blend easily.

3. Serve immediately with your strawberries by either drizzling the batter over the strawberries or using it as a dip. Alternatively, store in the refrigerator, where it will continue to thicken.

4. The batter can be kept in an airtight container in the refrigerator for up to 7 days.

Per serving (⅓ cup): Calories: 265; Fat: 6g; Carbohydrates: 48g; Fiber: 13g; Sugar: 19g; Protein: 11g; Sodium: 91mg

Cauliflower Buffalo Bites

These Buffalo bites are the perfect treat when you're craving something spicy and familiar. The flavor matches that of Buffalo wings, yet the cauliflower is filled with vitamins, fiber, and phytochemicals rather than poor-quality fats. Buy your cauliflower already prepared and cut into florets to make this quick and easy to prepare. Try dipping these bites in Ranch Dressing (page 184) for lick-your-fingers great flavor.

½ cup store-bought Buffalo wing sauce

1 tablespoon ghee

1 tablespoon coconut aminos

1 teaspoon apple cider vinegar

½ teaspoon garlic powder

1 large head cauliflower, stemmed and cut into florets

1. Preheat the oven to 425°F and line a baking sheet with parchment paper.

2. Place a small saucepan over medium heat and pour in the wing sauce, ghee, coconut aminos, vinegar, and garlic powder. When the ghee is melted, whisk well to combine.

3. In a large bowl, combine the cauliflower florets and ¼ cup of the Buffalo sauce. Toss to coat. Transfer the cauliflower to the baking sheet and bake for 17 to 20 minutes, tossing halfway through the baking time.

4. Transfer the wings to a serving dish and drizzle with the remaining ¼ cup of the Buffalo sauce. These are best served warm, but are just as good cold.

5. Store in an airtight container in the refrigerator for up to 7 days. Reheat in a 275°F oven for 10 minutes or in a microwave oven.

Per serving (1 cup): Calories: 89; Fat: 4g; Carbohydrates: 12g; Fiber: 5g; Sugar: 5g; Protein: 4g; Sodium: 181mg

- 30 MINUTES OR LESS
- NEXT-LEVEL ELIMINATION–FRIENDLY

Serves 4

Prep time: 10 minutes

Cook time: 20 minutes

Substitution Tip: If you are new to ghee, it is made from butter but the milk solids have been removed, leaving you with just the nutrient-rich fatty portion of the butter. If your supermarket doesn't carry it, the health food store will. You can also buy it online. If you are unable to find it, substitute avocado oil.

Cooking Tip: A good wing sauce is the key to this recipe. In my opinion, the best one is Frank's RedHot Buffalo wing sauce. It's clean, spicy, and flavorful.

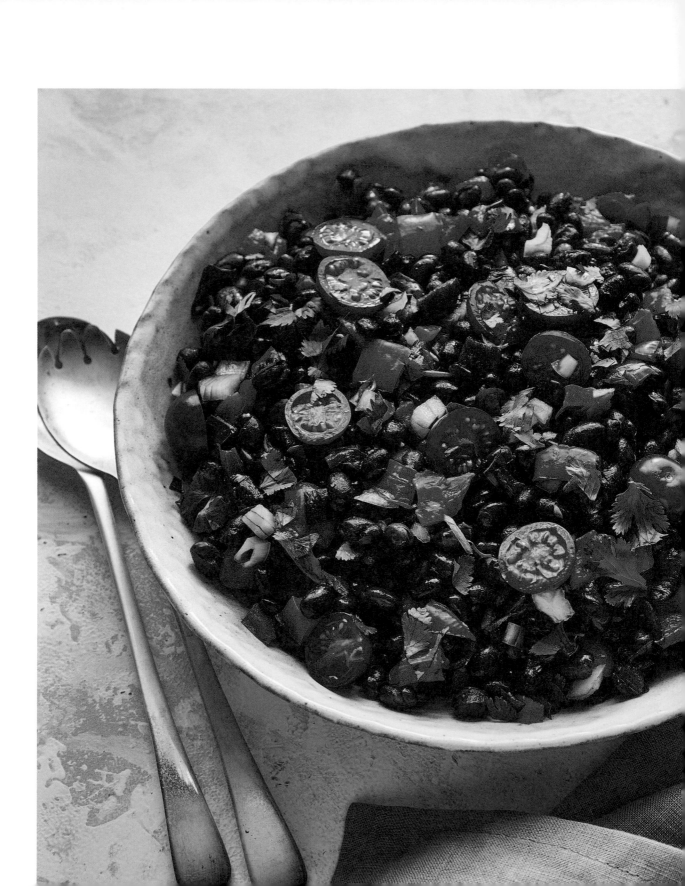

CHAPTER 7
Meatless Entrées

Curried Lentil Stew

This curried stew blends texture and flavor seamlessly. The acidity in the tomatoes tames the curry powder, and the soft texture of the cooked sweet potatoes makes them an ideal contrast to the lentils and cauliflower.

1 tablespoon avocado oil

1 medium onion, chopped

1 teaspoon garlic powder

2 tablespoons curry powder*

1 large or 2 small sweet potatoes, peeled and chopped

1 head cauliflower, stemmed and separated into bite-size florets

1 cup green lentils*

2 (14-ounce) cans diced tomatoes*

1 cup vegetable broth

1 teaspoon Himalayan or sea salt

1. In a 6-quart pot, heat the oil over medium heat. Add the onion and cook until softened and fragrant, about 5 minutes. Add the garlic powder and curry powder, making a paste. Stir constantly for 1 minute.

2. Stir in the sweet potatoes, cauliflower, lentils, tomatoes with their juices, and broth. Increase the heat to high. Bring to a boil, then reduce the heat to a simmer. Cover and cook until the lentils and sweet potatoes are tender, about 30 minutes.

3. Add the salt, stir well, and serve warm.

4. Once cooled, this soup can be stored in an airtight container in the refrigerator for up to 7 days or frozen in a zip-top bag for up to 6 months. Thaw completely in the refrigerator, then reheat in a saucepan on the stove.

Per serving (2 cups): Calories: 209; Fat: 4g; Carbohydrates: 35g; Fiber: 14g; Sugar: 7g; Protein: 12g; Sodium: 475mg

- ONE POT
- FREEZER-FRIENDLY

Serves 6

Prep time: 10 minutes

Cook time: 40 minutes

Time-Saving Tip: To save time prepping, buy the sweet potatoes already peeled and diced. You can also buy cauliflower stemmed and cut into florets. This makes it easier to just add to the pot.

Cooking Tip: This recipe can also be made in a slow cooker. Place all the ingredients in the slow cooker and cook on low for 4 hours or until the sweet potatoes and lentils are soft.

Sweet Potato Soup

Sweet potato soup is ideal for when you need a balanced meal in a hurry. The natural sweetness of sweet potatoes and coconut milk contrasts perfectly with the salt and spiciness of ginger, making it the perfect bowl of comfort food. Don't worry about how you chop the onions and sweet potatoes; they will all blend together in the end.

1 tablespoon avocado oil

1 small onion, roughly chopped

3 garlic cloves, minced

3 large sweet potatoes, peeled and roughly chopped

2 teaspoons ground ginger

2 cups vegetable broth

1 (14-ounce) can unsweetened, full-fat coconut milk

1 teaspoon Himalayan or sea salt

½ teaspoon black pepper* (optional)

1. Heat the oil in a 6-quart pot over medium heat. Add the onion and garlic and sauté for 5 minutes or until the onion pieces are golden brown and fragrant.

2. Add the sweet potatoes, ginger, broth, and coconut milk. Increase the heat to high and bring to a boil. Reduce the heat to low, cover, and let simmer until the sweet potatoes are soft, about 20 minutes. Add the salt and pepper (if using).

3. Using an immersion (handheld) blender, submerge the blender into the pot and blend the soup until it's creamy. Alternatively, allow the soup to cool slightly then transfer it to a blender and blend until pureed. You may have to do this in batches in a blender. Return to the pot and heat through. Serve warm.

4. Once cooled, this soup can be stored in an airtight container in the refrigerator for up to 7 days or frozen in a zip-top bag for up to 6 months. Thaw completely in the refrigerator, then reheat in a saucepan on the stove.

Per serving (1½ cups): Calories: 311; Fat: 22g; Carbohydrates: 26g; Fiber: 4g; Sugar: 5g; Protein: 6g; Sodium: 717mg

- ONE POT
- FREEZER-FRIENDLY
- NEXT-LEVEL ELIMINATION–FRIENDLY

Serves 4

Prep time: 10 minutes

Cook time: 30 minutes

Time-Saving Tip: Any time the oven is on, bake sweet potatoes and freeze them whole. Once thawed, they can be easily peeled and added to this soup to shorten the cook time. Alternatively, you can buy sweet potatoes already peeled and cubed.

Substitution Tip: This recipe works great with butternut squash as well, which can also be bought peeled and cubed for easy prep. For even richer flavor and to increase the anti-inflammatory properties, add 1 teaspoon of ground turmeric or cinnamon.

Fiesta Black Bean Salad

This is a hearty, sturdy salad that's full of nutrients. Bell peppers are a great source of vitamin C, which is necessary for thyroid hormone production, and the black beans are an excellent source of phytochemicals, fiber, and protein. Poblano peppers are milder than jalapeños, but they still have a bit of a kick. Their flavor becomes deep and rich when you roast them, as in this recipe.

For the salad

1 poblano pepper*

1 orange bell pepper*

1 yellow bell pepper*

1 small red onion

¼ cup fresh cilantro leaves

2 (14-ounce) cans black beans*, rinsed and drained

1 pint cherry tomatoes*

For the dressing

½ cup avocado oil

¼ cup balsamic vinegar

1 teaspoon Himalayan or sea salt

1 teaspoon white pepper* (optional)

1. Turn the oven to broil on low.

2. Core, seed, and cut the poblano pepper into quarters, then place on a baking sheet. Place the slices 6 to 8 inches away from the broiler and turn them every few minutes until they are lightly brown, about 12 minutes.

3. Core, seed, and dice the bell peppers. Dice the roasted poblano pepper and onion, cutting all about the same size as a black bean. Chop the cilantro. Set everything aside on your cutting board.

4. To make the dressing, in a large bowl whisk the oil, vinegar, salt, and white pepper (if using).

5. Add the peppers, onion, black beans, and cilantro and mix well.

6. Refrigerate for 2 hours or overnight to allow the flavors to meld.

7. Cut the cherry tomatoes in half and place on top just before serving.

8. Store in the refrigerator in an airtight container for up to 7 days.

Per serving (2 cups): Calories: 380; Fat: 28g; Carbohydrates: 27g; Fiber: 8g; Sugar: 7g; Protein: 8g; Sodium: 478mg

Serves 4

Prep time: 15 minutes, plus 2 hours to marinate

Cook time: 12 minutes

Cooking Tip: Roughly chop the onions and bell peppers, then place in a food processor for easier chopping.

Substitution Tip: This salad can be made with navy beans or garbanzo beans in place of the black beans.

Israeli Shakshuka

Shakshuka is a Middle Eastern dish consisting of eggs poached in a spicy tomato sauce. It can be served as breakfast, lunch, or dinner, and is a quick and easy meal to put together. The warm combination of spices is balanced by the subtle sweetness of honey. It is a delicious meal that always hits the spot.

1 tablespoon avocado oil

½ white onion, diced

2 garlic cloves, minced

1 red bell pepper*, seeded and diced

2 (14-ounce) cans diced tomatoes*

1 tablespoon tomato paste*

1 teaspoon chili powder*

1 teaspoon ground cumin*

1 teaspoon paprika*

1 teaspoon Himalayan or sea salt

1 teaspoon black pepper* (optional)

½ teaspoon cayenne pepper* (optional)

1 tablespoon honey

6 eggs*

Chopped fresh parsley

1. Heat the oil in a large sauté pan or skillet over medium heat. Add the onion and garlic and sauté until fragrant, about 5 minutes. Add the bell pepper, then stir and sauté for about 5 minutes.

2. Add the tomatoes, tomato paste, chili powder, cumin, paprika, salt, black pepper (if using), cayenne (if using), and honey to the pan. Stir well to incorporate and let simmer for 5 to 7 minutes.

3. Crack the eggs spaced evenly in the pan, cover, and let cook for 10 to 15 minutes, until the eggs are cooked to your liking.

4. Garnish with freshly chopped parsley and serve warm.

5. Shakshuka sauce can be stored in an airtight container in the refrigerator for up to 7 days. It can be heated on the stovetop when ready to use.

Per serving (2 eggs, 1 cup sauce): Calories: 257; Fat: 14g; Carbohydrates: 22g; Fiber: 5g; Sugar: 15g; Protein: 14g; Sodium: 1113mg

• ONE POT

Serves 3

Prep time: 10 minutes

Cook time: 30 minutes

Time-Saving Tip: Roughly chop the onions and bell pepper and put them in a food processor with the garlic. Using an S-blade, let the food processor do the work for you.

Caramelized Onion and Mushroom Spaghetti Squash

Mushrooms are one of the few foods with vitamin D, and there is a variety to choose from. White button and crimini mushrooms are similar, and have a mild flavor. Portobellos have a dense texture and rich flavor, while shiitakes have a meaty flavor. All of these, or a combination, work great for this recipe. The spaghetti squash here is an excellent nutrient-dense replacement for traditional spaghetti.

1 (2- to 3-pound) spaghetti squash

2 medium yellow onions

3 tablespoons ghee

1 pound mushrooms, sliced

1 cup chopped kale

¼ cup chopped fresh parsley

½ teaspoon Himalayan or sea salt

¼ teaspoon black pepper* (optional)

1. Preheat the oven to 400°F.

2. Slice the squash in half, scrape out the seeds, and place cut side down on a baking dish. Roast for 35 to 45 minutes. When you can pierce the outside with a fork, it is done.

3. While the squash is roasting, cut the onions into long strips.

4. Melt the ghee over medium heat in a large sauté pan or skillet, then add the onions, stirring occasionally as they start caramelizing. After 5 minutes, add the mushrooms, then the kale. Cook together until the onions turn golden brown, about 10 minutes more.

5. When the squash is cooked, remove it from the oven and allow to cool. When it's cool enough to handle, use the tines of a fork to "spaghetti" (scrape) the squash into the skillet with the onion mixture. Add the parsley, salt, and pepper (if using) and stir everything together over medium heat to warm through. Serve as you would a spaghetti dish.

6. Store in an airtight container in the refrigerator for up to 7 days. Reheat in a saucepan on the stove or in the microwave oven in a bowl.

Per serving (2 cups): Calories: 187; Fat: 11g; Carbohydrates: 21g; Fiber: 3g; Sugar: 4g; Protein: 6g; Sodium: 278mg

- 5 INGREDIENT OR LESS
- NEXT-LEVEL ELIMINATION–FRIENDLY

Serves 4

Prep time: 15 minutes, plus time to cool

Cook time: 50 minutes

Time-Saving Tip: Cook the spaghetti squash another day, perhaps when you have the oven on for something else. After cooking and cooling, both halves can be stored in the refrigerator for up to 5 days before preparing the "spaghetti."

Cooking Tip: To make the spaghetti squash easier to cut, microwave it whole on high for 2 minutes. This will soften the tough, outer skin, making it easier to pierce with a knife.

Seven Vegetable Soup

This soup is a staple you'll want to always have on hand. The ginger is spicy while being gentle on your stomach, and the turnips are a good replacement for the potatoes in traditional vegetable soup.

1 tablespoon
  avocado oil

2 large onions, chopped

2 stalks celery, chopped

6 cups vegetable broth

3 cups chopped kale

3 small
  zucchini; chopped

1 pound
  mushrooms, sliced

2 turnips, peeled
  and chopped

4 carrots, shredded

½ cup chopped
  fresh parsley

1 teaspoon
  ground ginger

1 teaspoon Himalayan or
  sea salt

½ teaspoon black
  pepper* (optional)

- ONE POT
- FREEZER-FRIENDLY
- NEXT-LEVEL
  ELIMINATION–FRIENDLY

Serves 6

Prep time: 15 minutes

Cook time: 30 minutes

Time-Saving Tip: You can buy chopped onions, chopped kale, sliced mushrooms, and carrot sticks to reduce the prep time for this soup.

Substitution Tip: You can add other vegetables to this soup or substitute any with greens (collard greens, mustard greens, beet greens, or Swiss chard), shaved Brussels sprouts, cabbage, or coleslaw mix.

1. Heat the oil in a 6-quart pot over medium heat. Add the onions and celery and sauté for 5 minutes.

2. Add the broth, kale, zucchini, mushrooms, and turnips. Cover and simmer for 20 minutes.

3. Add the carrots, parsley, ginger, salt, and pepper (if using). Cover and simmer for 5 minutes. Serve warm.

4. Once cooled, store in an airtight container in the refrigerator for up to 7 days or frozen in a zip-top bag for up to 6 months. Thaw completely in the refrigerator, then reheat in a saucepan on the stove.

Per serving (2 cups): Calories: 153; Fat: 4g; Carbohydrates: 21g; Fiber: 5g; Sugar: 9g; Protein: 10g; Sodium: 732mg

Shaved Brussels Sprouts and Apple Salad

This salad is super crunchy thanks to the perfect blend of ingredients—Brussels sprouts, pumpkin and sunflower seeds, and apples. The pumpkin seeds are an excellent source of zinc and tyrosine, and a plant-based source of iron—all necessary for proper thyroid hormone production. As quick as this salad is to prepare, you can make it even quicker by buying shaved Brussels sprouts in the refrigerated section of the grocery store.

1 pound
    Brussels sprouts

½ red onion, chopped

1 small apple, cored
    and chopped

⅓ cup raisins

¼ cup sunflower seeds*

⅓ cup pumpkin seeds*

Balsamic Vinaigrette
    (page 182)

1. Trim and discard any loose leaves from the Brussels sprouts. Cut the Brussels sprouts in half, then shred them using the S-blade of a food processor, or thinly slice them with a knife. Set aside.

2. Mix the Brussels sprouts, red onion, chopped apple, raisins, sunflower seeds, and pumpkin seeds. Toss with the vinaigrette and serve cold.

3. Store in an airtight container in the refrigerator for up to 5 days.

Per serving (2 cups): Calories: 345; Fat: 21g; Carbohydrates: 33g; Fiber: 8g; Sugar: 17g; Protein: 10g; Sodium: 136mg

• **30 MINUTES OR LESS**

Serves 4

Prep time: 10 minutes

Next-Level Elimination Tip: If nuts and seeds are a problem for you, just leave them out of this salad. It will still have plenty of flavor and crunch.

Time-Saving Tip: You can use store-bought balsamic vinaigrette salad dressing. Be careful to look for a dressing made with avocado, olive, safflower, or sunflower oil, such as Primal Kitchen Balsamic Vinaigrette and Marinade, or one of Sir Kensington's vinaigrettes, such as Golden Citrus.

Samosa-Inspired Veggie Casserole

This veggie casserole is inspired by Indian samosas. I've kept all the delicious filling, but left out the glutenous dough. The turmeric adds a beautiful golden color, making it appealing to the eye, and the flavors will explode in your mouth, making this dish one you will crave.

1 tablespoon avocado oil

1 onion, chopped

2 large turnips, peeled and cubed

3 garlic cloves, minced

2 medium carrots, chopped

1 cup frozen peas*

3 tablespoons vegetable broth or water

½ teaspoon ground ginger

1 teaspoon garam masala*

¼ teaspoon black pepper* (optional)

½ teaspoon ground turmeric

½ teaspoon Himalayan or sea salt

4 cups fresh spinach

1. Preheat the oven to 375°F. Grease a 10-by-13-inch baking dish.

2. In a 4-quart pot, heat the oil over medium heat, then add the onion pieces and cook until they caramelize, about 5 minutes.

3. Add the turnips, garlic, carrots, peas, broth, ginger, garam masala, pepper (if using), turmeric, and salt and stir well. Cook for about 10 minutes.

4. Add this mixture to the prepared baking dish and bake for 15 minutes, or until the casserole is browned on top. Serve hot over a bed of fresh spinach. The heat from the casserole will wilt the spinach.

5. Store in an airtight container in the refrigerator for up to 7 days. This would be a great recipe to double and freeze as a whole casserole. To reheat, thaw completely in the refrigerator, then bake at 375°F for 25 to 30 minutes or until it's bubbling on top.

Per serving (1½ cups): Calories: 117; Fat: 4g; Carbohydrates: 18g; Fiber: 5g; Sugar: 7g; Protein: 4g; Sodium: 386mg

• FREEZER-FRIENDLY

Serves 4

Prep time: 10 minutes

Cook time: 30 minutes

Time-Saving Tip: To save time prepping, buy chopped onions, shredded carrots, and minced garlic.

Substitution Tip: Garam masala is a spice blend, usually of cumin, coriander, green and black cardamom, cinnamon, nutmeg, cloves, bay leaves, peppercorns, fennel, mace, and dried chilies. If you can't find it, you can substitute curry powder, or make your own blend.

Coconut Curry over Cauliflower Rice

Riced cauliflower makes a great substitute for rice, and also adds a vegetable into the mix. When making riced cauliflower, resist the urge to steam it and instead brown and crisp it on the stove, making the texture more like rice. Then you can drown it in the delectable coconut curry.

1 tablespoon avocado oil

1 onion, chopped

4 garlic cloves, minced

1 teaspoon ground ginger

1 tablespoon ground turmeric

2 large zucchini, diced

1 pound mushrooms, chopped

1 (14-ounce) can unsweetened, full-fat coconut milk

1 teaspoon Himalayan or sea salt

1 cup Cauliflower Rice (page 177)

1. In a 4-quart pot, heat the oil over medium-high heat. Add the onion and stir well. Cook for 5 to 7 minutes until it starts to caramelize.

2. Add the garlic, ginger, and turmeric and stir well, making a paste. Cook for 1 to 2 minutes until it becomes fragrant. Add the zucchini and mushrooms, and cook until golden brown, for 3 to 5 minutes.

3. Pour in the coconut milk and salt. Increase the heat to high, bring to a boil, then reduce to a simmer. Cook until the liquid reduces and thickens, for 5 to 7 minutes, stirring frequently.

4. Serve the coconut curry over the cauliflower rice.

5. Store in an airtight container in the refrigerator for up to 5 days. Reheat in a saucepan on the stove.

Per serving (1½ cups, ½ cup cauliflower rice): Calories: 692; Fat: 50g; Carbohydrates: 56g; Fiber: 19g; Sugar: 22g; Protein: 25g; Sodium: 937mg

- NEXT-LEVEL ELIMINATION–FRIENDLY

Serves 2

Prep time: 15 minutes

Cook time: 20 minutes

Substitution Tip: Instead of using zucchini, you can substitute 1 medium eggplant, which has a hearty texture and absorbs the curry flavors like a sponge. Peeling is optional.

Time-Saving Tip: You can buy chopped onions and minced garlic to save on prep time.

Stuffed Portobello Burgers

Portobello mushrooms have a hearty, meaty texture and absorb marinade like a sponge. Mushrooms are high in vitamin D, and bell peppers are one of the highest sources of vitamin C, both of which are necessary for producing thyroid hormone.

4 portobello mushrooms

½ cup balsamic vinegar

2 tablespoons avocado oil, divided

2 tablespoons coconut aminos

2 teaspoons dried basil

2 teaspoons dried oregano

2 teaspoons minced garlic

½ teaspoon white pepper* (optional)

1 red onion, sliced

2 bell peppers*, any colors, seeded and sliced

3 cups fresh spinach, cut into small pieces

1 teaspoon Himalayan or sea salt

1. Remove the stems from the mushrooms and wipe the caps clean with a paper towel. Don't rinse with water, as it will alter the texture as the mushroom cooks.

2. Place the mushrooms smooth-side down in a baking dish or on a plate.

3. In a small bowl, whisk together the vinegar, 1 tablespoon of oil, coconut aminos, basil, oregano, garlic, and white pepper (if using). Pour the marinade over the mushrooms and let marinate for at least 30 minutes.

4. While the mushrooms are marinating, slice the onion and bell peppers.

5. In a heavy cast iron pan or a grill pan, cook the mushrooms over medium heat, using the excess marinade to baste as they are cooking. Cook for 5 to 8 minutes on each side.

6. In a separate sauté pan, combine the remaining 1 tablespoon of oil, onion, and bell peppers and sauté over medium heat for about 10 minutes, until the onion starts to caramelize. Add the spinach and salt and stir until the spinach begins to wilt, about 3 minutes. Stuff the mushrooms with the spinach stuffing and serve warm.

7. Store in an airtight container in the refrigerator for up to 5 days. Reheat by placing in an oven or toaster oven at 275°F, or in a microwave oven on a plate.

Per serving: Calories: 150; Fat: 7g; Carbohydrates: 17g; Fiber: 3g; Sugar: 9g; Protein: 5g; Sodium: 496mg

Serves 4

Prep time: 10 minutes, plus 30 minutes to marinate

Cook time: 20 minutes

Cooking Tip: You can start these mushrooms marinating before you leave for work in the morning. They will absorb the flavors all day, making them perfect and ready when you are.

Next-Level Elimination Tip: While bell peppers are a great source of vitamin C, they are also nightshade vegetables and the natural solanine could potentially be a triggering ingredient. You can eliminate the peppers and replace them with diced carrots.

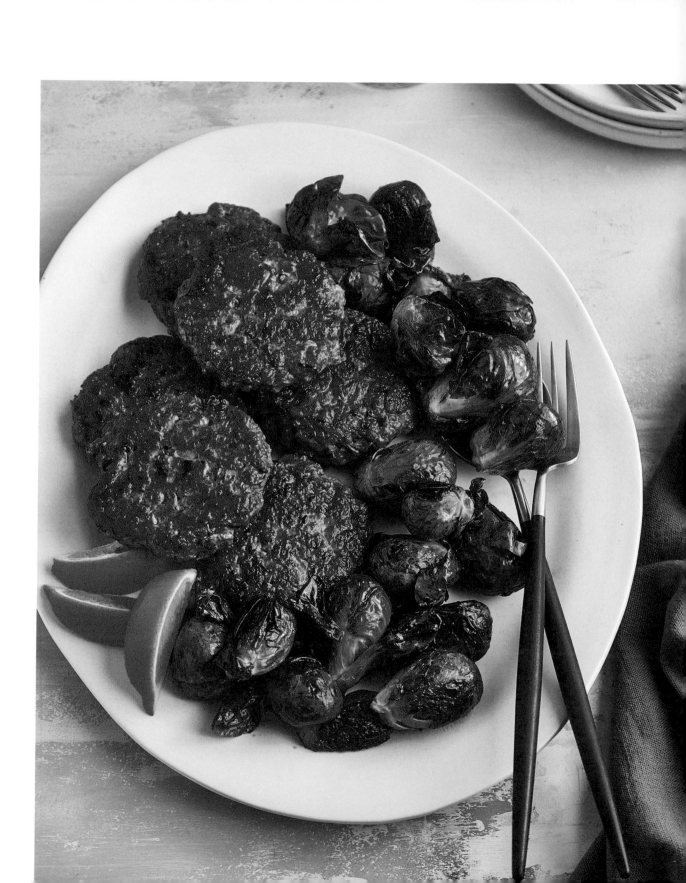

CHAPTER 8
Seafood Entrées

Crunchy Tuna Salad

Canned tuna can be a simple way to eat healthy fish and omega-3 fats. But be careful when buying canned tuna, as it is often packed in vegetable broth or oil, both of which usually contain soy. Tuna packed in low-sodium broth or water usually will have no soy, but be sure to read the ingredient labels carefully.

2 (5-ounce) cans tuna packed in low-sodium broth or water

½ apple, cored and diced

2 stalks celery, sliced

½ small red onion, diced

1 avocado, pitted and sliced

½ teaspoon Himalayan or sea salt

¼ teaspoon black pepper* (optional)

2 tablespoons Citrus Ginger Cilantro Dressing (page 183)

Juice of 1 lime or 1 tablespoon lime juice (optional)

- ONE POT
- 30 MINUTES OR LESS
- NEXT-LEVEL ELIMINATION–FRIENDLY

Serves 2

Prep time: 10 minutes

Substitution Tip: Feel free to substitute canned salmon in place of tuna. And if you'd prefer a store-bought dressing, Primal Kitchen's Sesame Ginger Vinaigrette and Marinade is made with avocado oil (rather than the soybean oil in most salad dressings) and is a good choice.

Cooking Tip: If you plan to save some of this salad for later, adding the lime juice will help preserve the avocado and prevent it from turning brown.

1. Drain the cans of tuna and break up the fish in a medium bowl. Add the apple, celery, red onion, avocado, salt, and pepper (if using).

2. If eating immediately, top with the dressing, toss, and serve.

3. If preparing in advance to serve later, squeeze the lime juice on top of the tuna salad, mix gently, and cover. Store in an airtight container in the refrigerator for up to 3 days. Toss with the dressing before serving.

Per serving: Calories: 431; Fat: 21g; Carbohydrates: 18g; Fiber: 9g; Sugar: 8g; Protein: 44g; Sodium: 583mg

Ginger-Spiced Tuna Salad Wraps

The many flavors and textures of this tuna salad will leave you wanting more. The slight crunch of lettuce and onions perfectly matches with the smoothness of the tuna, while the ginger provides just the kick it needs to make you feel satisfied. If you love salmon more than tuna, substitute canned salmon for tuna. Be sure to check the ingredients on either one to make sure there is no soy in the broth.

2 (5-ounce) cans tuna packed in low-sodium broth or water

½ small red onion, finely diced

2 scallions, sliced

½ teaspoon ground ginger

¼ cup Homemade Healthy Mayonnaise* (page 181)

8 leaves butter leaf lettuce or Romaine lettuce

1. Drain the can of tuna and break up the fish in a medium bowl. Add the onion, scallions, ginger, and mayonnaise and stir well to combine.

2. Refrigerate for 20 minutes, or until thoroughly chilled.

3. Spoon into lettuce leaves and serve.

4. The stuffing for this recipe can be doubled and stored in an airtight container in the refrigerator for up to 3 days.

Per serving (4 wraps): Calories: 229; Fat: 15g; Carbohydrates: 2g; Fiber: 1g; Sugar: 1g; Protein: 22g; Sodium: 109mg

• **ONE POT**

Serves 2

Prep time: 10 minutes, plus 20 minutes to chill

Substitution Tip: If you would prefer a store-bought mayonnaise, Hain Pure Foods mayonnaise is made with safflower oil and Sir Kensington's mayonnaise is made with avocado oil; both are good alternatives.

Cooking Tip: This recipe is written very simply, but you can dress it up by adding ¼ cup chopped fresh cilantro, 1 teaspoon red chili paste, minced jalapeño peppers, and sesame seeds. Get creative and explore the flavors you enjoy.

Shrimp and Veggie Stir-Fry

Stir-fry is a great recipe to fall back on when you need a quick, nourishing, and complete meal. The broccoli here is a great source of vitamin C, which aids with the production of thyroid hormone. Most store-bought stir-fry sauces are made with soy sauce, which is why I recommend using the homemade version here. It will keep in the refrigerator for a month.

1 pound shrimp, peeled and deveined

⅓ cup Stir-Fry Sauce* (page 187)

2 tablespoons sesame oil*, divided

1 small onion, sliced

1 small head cabbage, sliced

3 cups broccoli, cut into bite-size florets

1 tablespoon toasted sesame seeds*

1. Place the shrimp and stir-fry sauce in a small mixing bowl. Let marinate for about 20 minutes on the counter, or in the refrigerator for up to 4 hours.

2. To make the stir-fry, heat 1 tablespoon of sesame oil in a skillet or wok over medium-high heat. Add the onion and sauté for 5 minutes, or until fragrant and translucent.

3. Add the remaining 1 tablespoon of sesame oil, cabbage, and broccoli and sauté for about 5 minutes more, until the cabbage begins to wilt and the broccoli begins to soften.

4. Pour the shrimp and marinade into the skillet. Stir until the sauce coats the shrimp and vegetables. Stir-fry for 5 to 7 minutes, or until the shrimp turns pink and slightly opaque with a little white. Top with toasted sesame seeds and serve.

5. Store in an airtight container in the refrigerator for up to 3 days. Reheat by warming in a skillet on the stove or in a bowl in the microwave.

Per serving (2 cups): Calories: 305; Fat: 13g; Carbohydrates: 23g; Fiber: 7g; Sugar: 8g; Protein: 28g; Sodium: 393mg

Serves 4

Prep time: 15 minutes, plus 20 minutes or more to marinate

Cook time: 15 minutes

Time-Saving Tip: Rather than buying a whole head of cabbage, buy coleslaw mix, which is shredded green and red cabbage mixed with some shredded carrots. This will save the time and mess of cutting up a whole cabbage.

Next-Level Elimination Tip: Since seeds can potentially be a triggering ingredient, use avocado oil instead of sesame oil and omit the sesame seed garnish.

Shrimp Curry

This one-pot meal is always a crowd pleaser. Just when you think it might be spicy, the ginger comes to the rescue and soothes the palate. Ginger is also very soothing for the gastrointestinal tract and helps calm inflammation—an added bonus. Serve this dish in bowls as a stew, or over Cauliflower Rice (page 177). This recipe is a great one to double, giving you leftovers to freeze.

2 tablespoons avocado oil, divided

½ onion, thinly sliced

2 garlic cloves, minced

2 teaspoons ground ginger

4 tablespoons red curry paste*

1 large head broccoli, cut into florets

1 large sweet potato, peeled and cubed

1 (14-ounce) can diced tomatoes*

1 (14-ounce) can unsweetened, full-fat coconut milk

½ teaspoon cayenne pepper* (optional)

1 teaspoon Himalayan or sea salt

Juice of 1 lemon or 2 tablespoons lemon juice

1 pound shrimp, peeled and deveined

1. In a Dutch oven or stockpot, heat 1 tablespoon of avocado oil over medium-high heat. Add the onion, garlic, and ginger and sauté until fragrant, about 5 minutes.

2. Add the remaining 1 tablespoon of avocado oil, curry paste, broccoli, sweet potato, and canned tomatoes with their juices, and sauté for about 5 minutes. Add the coconut milk and stir to combine.

3. Add the cayenne (if using), salt, and lemon juice. Increase the heat to high and bring the mixture to a boil. Reduce the heat to medium, cover, and let cook for 30 minutes, stirring periodically.

4. Add the shrimp and uncover the pot so some of the moisture can evaporate. Cook uncovered for about 10 minutes. Serve immediately.

5. Once cooled, this curry can be stored in an airtight container in the refrigerator for up to 4 days or frozen in a zip-top bag for up to 6 months. When ready to eat, thaw in the refrigerator, then warm the contents in a saucepan on the stove.

Per serving (1½ cups): Calories: 369; Fat: 24g; Carbohydrates: 19g; Fiber: 3g; Sugar: 5g; Protein: 21g; Sodium: 1143mg

- ONE POT
- FREEZER-FRIENDLY

Serves 6

Prep time: 15 minutes

Cook time: 50 minutes

Substitution Tip: If you can get crawfish, they make a great substitute for shrimp in this recipe.

Time-Saving Tip: Buy precut sweet potatoes and broccoli in the produce section to make prep time a bit easier.

Spicy Shrimp, Okra, and Tomato Stew

This recipe is simple to prepare, yet it tastes like you worked hard in the kitchen all day. It's a good representation of Creole cooking, with the combination of okra and tomatoes. The shrimp also provides an excellent source of protein and iodine, important for building thyroid hormones. Serve this dish in bowls as a stew, or over Cauliflower Rice (page 177).

1 tablespoon avocado oil

1 onion, chopped

1 medium jalapeño pepper*, seeded and minced (optional)

2 pounds okra, sliced into ½-inch pieces

3 (14-ounce) cans stewed tomatoes*

½ cup seafood stock or vegetable broth

1 bay leaf

1 teaspoon Himalayan or sea salt

2 pounds shrimp, peeled and deveined

1. In a Dutch oven or stockpot, heat the avocado oil over medium-high heat. Add the onion and jalapeño (if using) and sauté until golden brown, about 5 minutes.

2. Add the okra and sauté until it starts to soften, another 5 minutes.

3. Add the tomatoes with their juices, stock, bay leaf, and salt. Increase the heat to high. Bring to a boil, then reduce the heat, cover, and simmer for about 15 minutes, until the okra is tender.

4. Remove the cover and increase the heat to medium. Add the shrimp and cook until the liquid thickens and the shrimp turns pink and opaque with a little white, for 5 to 7 minutes. Serve immediately.

5. Once cooled, this stew can be stored in an air-tight container in the refrigerator for up to 4 days or frozen in a zip-top bag for up to 6 months. When ready to eat, thaw in the refrigerator, then warm the contents in a saucepan on the stove.

Per serving (1½ cups): Calories: 257; Fat: 4g; Carbohydrates: 21g; Fiber: 8g; Sugar: 8g; Protein: 36g; Sodium: 506mg

- ONE POT
- FREEZER-FRIENDLY

Serves 6

Prep time: 15 minutes

Cook time: 30 minutes

Time-Saving Tip: You can buy frozen okra already sliced. If you let it thaw, it won't change the cook time. If you add it frozen, it will take about 10 minutes more to cook in step 3.

Cooking Tip: Shrimp cooks quickly. You'll know it's cooked when it turns from gray to pink, and is slightly opaque and a little white. Be careful to not overcook the shrimp because it will make it tough and rubbery.

Shrimp Cauliflower Fried Rice

This recipe is (an almost) classic shrimp fried rice. By replacing the rice with cauliflower, you prevent the rapid rise of blood sugar. This dish is also packed with iodine and selenium from the shrimp and vitamin A from the carrots, both of which help promote the production of thyroid hormone.

2 tablespoons
  sesame oil*

1 medium
  onion, chopped

4 garlic cloves, minced

4 cups Cauliflower Rice
  (page 177)

1 pound shrimp, peeled
  and deveined

2 medium carrots,
  shredded

1 cup green peas*

4 eggs*

- ONE POT

Serves 4

Prep time: 15 minutes

Cook time: 10 minutes

Next-Level Elimination Tip: Although eggs are an excellent source of protein, they are also a common food sensitivity. If you need to eliminate them, simply add 8 more ounces of shrimp.

Substitution Tip: Feel free to get creative with the vegetables used in this recipe. Other vegetables that go great with fried rice are snow peas, chopped asparagus, broccoli, and bell peppers. Choose the ones you enjoy most.

1. In a wok or a large skillet, heat the sesame oil over medium-high heat. Add the onion and garlic and cook for 3 to 5 minutes.

2. Add the cauliflower rice and shrimp, then stir and cook for 1 minute. Add the carrots and peas, then stir and cook for 3 minutes.

3. Clear a circle in the center of the pan and crack in the eggs. Stir to scramble the eggs and combine them with the other ingredients. Cook until the eggs are fully cooked, about 3 minutes. Serve immediately.

4. Store this in an airtight container in the refrigerator for up to 3 days. Reheat in a skillet on the stove or in a bowl in the microwave.

Per serving (2 cups): Calories: 305; Fat: 13g; Carbohydrates: 17g; Fiber: 6g; Sugar: 8g; Protein: 33g; Sodium: 246mg

White Fish Red Curry

Cooking fish can be tricky, but tossing it in a stew makes it much easier to master. The cauliflower rice adds texture, and curry paste provides a great flavor kick. Cod is a good source of tyrosine, which is the backbone of building all thyroid hormones, making this dish nutrient-dense and very satisfying.

1 tablespoon
   avocado oil

1 large onion, diced

2 garlic cloves, minced

2 tablespoons red
   curry paste*

2 (14-ounce) cans
   diced tomatoes*

1 cup vegetable broth
   or seafood stock

4 (6-ounce) cod fillets

2 cups Cauliflower Rice
   (page 177)

- ONE POT

Serves 4

Prep time: 5 minutes

Cook time: 20 minutes

Substitution Tip: Instead of cod, other white, flaky fish you can use in this recipe are bass, grouper, or snapper.

Cooking Tip: The thickness of the fish will dictate how quickly it cooks. A thin fillet may cook in 7 to 9 minutes, while a thick one may take as long as 15 minutes. Keep this in mind when you are cooking. Also, stirring too frequently after the fish is cooked will cause it to fall apart.

1. In a Dutch oven or stockpot, heat the avocado oil on medium-high heat. Add the onion and garlic and sauté for about 5 minutes, until soft and fragrant.

2. Add the curry paste and stir for 1 to 2 minutes, then add the tomatoes with their juices and the stock. Bring to a simmer.

3. When the mixture is simmering, gently add the fish and cook for 10 to 12 minutes, or until the fish flakes easily. Serve immediately over cauliflower rice.

4. Store this curry in an airtight container in the refrigerator for up to 3 days. Reheat in a saucepan on the stove or in a bowl in a microwave oven.

Per serving (½ cup cauliflower rice, 12 ounces stew):
Calories: 294; Fat: 8g; Carbohydrates: 21g; Fiber: 7g;
Sugar: 11g; Protein: 36g; Sodium: 640mg

Salmon Rosemary Patties with Roasted Brussels Sprouts

Salmon is a great source of omega-3 fats, which can help to calm inflammation. Whether you are using fresh salmon or canned, it has healing properties and tastes delicious. Paired with the Brussels sprouts, a great source of vitamin C that is useful for hormone production, this is a truly nutrient-dense meal. Serve with lemon wedges, if desired.

For the Brussels sprouts

1½ pounds Brussels sprouts

2 tablespoons avocado oil

½ teaspoon Himalayan or sea salt

½ teaspoon black pepper* (optional)

For the salmon patties

6 scallions, roughly chopped

1 tablespoon roughly chopped fresh rosemary

1 teaspoon seasoning blend or seafood seasoning blend

½ teaspoon black pepper* (optional)

1½ pounds salmon fillet, skin removed

1 tablespoon avocado oil

1. Preheat the oven to 400°F and line a baking sheet with parchment paper.

2. Trim off the stem ends of the Brussels sprouts, cut off any brown spots, and pull off any loose outer leaves. Discard these trimmings.

3. In a large bowl, mix the Brussels sprouts with the avocado oil, salt, and pepper (if using). Spread them on the baking sheet in a single layer.

4. Bake for 35 to 40 minutes, until crisp on the outside and tender on the inside. Serve warm.

5. Store the cooked Brussels sprouts in an airtight container in the refrigerator for up to 7 days. Reheat in a skillet or microwave.

6. While the Brussels sprouts are roasting, place the scallions, rosemary, seasoning blend, and black pepper (if using) in a food processor fitted with an S-blade and pulse until minced.

7. Add half the salmon and process again until the salmon is ground. Use a spatula to scrape down the sides, then add the rest of the salmon and process until everything is ground and the mixture begins to form a ball.

8. Using wet hands, form the mixture into 6 patties.

9. Heat a sauté pan or skillet over medium heat. Heat the avocado oil, then place 3 patties in the pan, cook for about 4 minutes, then gently flip and cook for 4 minutes more. Repeat with the remaining patties. Plate the salmon patties with the Brussels sprouts and serve warm.

10. Salmon patties can be stored in an airtight container for up to 4 days or frozen. Place them in a zip-top bag in the freezer, where they will keep for 3 months. When ready to eat, thaw in the refrigerator, then reheat on medium-low heat in a skillet on the stove.

Per serving (1 salmon patty, ½ cup Brussels sprouts):
Calories: 316; Fat: 19g; Carbohydrates: 12g; Fiber: 5g; Sugar: 3g; Protein: 26g; Sodium: 252mg

- FREEZER-FRIENDLY
- NEXT-LEVEL ELIMINATION–FRIENDLY

Serves 6

Prep time: 15 minutes

Cook time: 40 minutes

Substitution Tip: Roasted broccoli also works great with this recipe. Roast the broccoli the same way as the Brussels sprouts, but decrease the time to 25 minutes.

Cooking Tip: You can also use 2 (14-ounce) cans of salmon for this recipe. Canned salmon sometimes has soft, fragile bones. These bones do not have to be removed and can be processed into the patties in the food processor. They are so soft that once processed you won't even know they are there. They are an excellent source of calcium.

Chili-Glazed Salmon with Roasted Veggies

The combination of flavors here is explosive in your mouth. The texture of salmon with the slight crunch of the vegetables pairs perfectly with a baked sweet potato. Salmon is a great source of omega-3 fatty acids, and when combined with ginger it is helpful for decreasing general inflammation that is common with Hashimoto's.

For the salmon and veggies

4 (6-ounce) salmon fillets

1 red bell pepper*, seeded and sliced

1 yellow bell pepper*, seeded and sliced

1 onion, sliced

4 carrots, sliced

1 medium sweet potato, peeled and diced

For the marinade

½ cup sweet Thai chili sauce*

¼ cup coconut aminos

2 teaspoons ground ginger

1 tablespoon lime juice

1. Preheat the oven to 375°F and line a baking sheet with parchment paper.

2. Lay the salmon skin-side down on the baking sheet, surrounded by the bell peppers, onion, carrots, and sweet potato.

3. To make the marinade, in a small bowl, whisk together the Thai chili sauce, coconut aminos, ginger, and lime juice. Drizzle ¾ of the marinade over the salmon and vegetables, reserving ¼ of the marinade for later.

4. Cover the pan with foil and bake for 10 minutes. Remove the foil and broil on low for 5 minutes more, until the top of the fish starts to blacken.

5. Remove the baking sheet from the oven and brush the remaining ¼ of the marinade over the salmon. Serve each fillet of salmon with the veggies and sweet potatoes on the side.

6. Store in an airtight container in the refrigerator for up to 3 days. Reheat in the oven or toaster oven at 275°F, or in a skillet on the stove over medium heat.

Per serving (1 fish fillet, 1½ cups veggies): Calories: 427; Fat: 12g; Carbohydrates: 38g; Fiber: 4g; Sugar: 21g; Protein: 41g; Sodium: 771mg

• **30 MINUTES OR LESS**

Serves 4

Prep time: 10 minutes

Cook time: 15 minutes

Time-Saving Tip: Buy peeled and cut sweet potatoes in the refrigerated produce section of the grocery store. When purchased this way, use half the bag in this recipe.

Cooking Tip: To ensure that the carrots and sweet potatoes cook completely, cut them into small pieces. Sweet potatoes should not be larger than gaming dice and carrot slices no thicker than two nickels.

Poached Cod with Summer Vegetables and Quinoa

Cod is a white, flaky fish with a very mild flavor. It's a great source of iodine, which is essential for thyroid hormone development. With the combination of quinoa and vegetables, this dish offers a variety of tastes and textures for your palate to enjoy.

For the quinoa

1 cup quinoa*

2 cups water or broth

¼ teaspoon Himalayan or sea salt

For the fish and veggies

2 tablespoons avocado oil

1 small red onion, sliced

1 fennel bulb, cut in half and sliced

2 medium zucchini, cut into
   ½-inch pieces

5 Roma tomatoes*, diced

4 (6-ounce) cod fillets

2 teaspoons Italian seasoning

½ teaspoon Himalayan or sea salt

¼ teaspoon black pepper* (optional)

To make the quinoa

1. Pour the quinoa into a fine mesh colander and rinse under running water for at least 30 seconds, then drain well. This removes the bitter outer coating.

2. In a 2-quart saucepan, bring the water, rinsed quinoa, and salt to a boil over medium-high. Reduce the heat to low and maintain a gentle simmer. Cook the quinoa for about 10 minutes, or until it's absorbed all the water.

3. Remove from the heat, cover, and let the quinoa sit for 5 minutes.

To make the fish and veggies

1. While the quinoa is cooking, heat the oil in a large sauté pan or skillet over medium heat. Add the onion and sauté for 5 minutes or until fragrant and soft. Add the fennel, zucchini, and tomatoes and sauté for 5 to 7 minutes more. Remove the veggies from the skillet and set aside.

2. Season the fish with Italian seasoning, salt, and pepper (if using). Using the same skillet the veggies were cooked in, pour 2 cups of water into the pan and heat until the water is starting to bubble on the sides. Add the fish, cover, and poach at a low simmer for 10 to 12 minutes, depending on the thickness of your fish.

3. Remove the fish with a slotted spatula. Serve the fish with the veggies and a side of quinoa.

4. Store in an airtight container in the refrigerator for up to 3 days. Reheat the fish in an oven on 275°F for 10 to 15 minutes. Reheat the veggies and quinoa in a skillet on the stove or a bowl in the microwave.

Per serving (1 fillet, 1 cup veggies): Calories: 422; Fat: 12g; Carbohydrates: 42g; Fiber: 8g; Sugar: 7g; Protein: 39g; Sodium: 507mg

Serves 4

Prep time: 15 minutes

Cook time: 25 minutes

Substitution Tip: Swap the vegetables for anything seasonal, including yellow squash, broccoli, or halved Brussels sprouts. Additionally, the cod can be replaced with halibut, snapper, bass, or grouper.

Cooking Tip: The temperature of the water when poaching fish is important. It should be just hot enough to start bubbling only on the sides of the pan. Do not allow the water to start boiling, as that will cook the outside of the fish but not cook it all the way through.

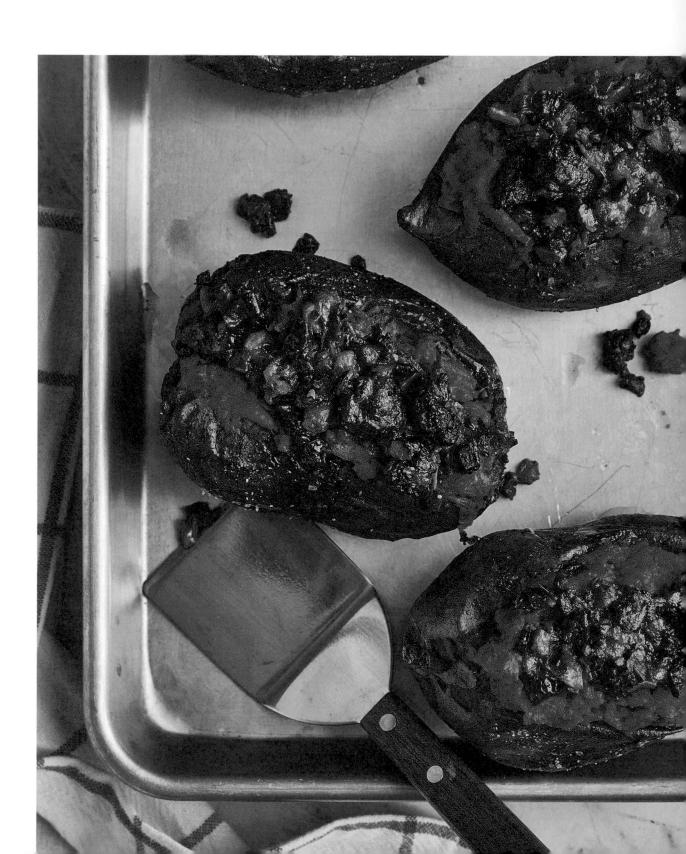

CHAPTER 9
Poultry and Meat Entrées

Nutty Chicken Lettuce Wraps

This is a quick and easy meal that can be made for nearly a week's worth of lunches. Butter lettuce is a soft, pliable lettuce that is a good replacement for tortillas, or you can use Plantain Tortillas (page 178). The crunch of the cucumber and onion complements the creaminess of the Cashew Sauce (page 188).

1 cooked rotisserie chicken, bones and skin removed (about 3 cups)

1 medium cucumber, chopped

½ small red onion, finely diced

¾ cup Cashew Sauce* (page 188)

12 butter lettuce or Romaine leaves

- ONE POT
- 5 INGREDIENTS OR LESS
- 30 MINUTES OR LESS

Serves 6

Prep time: 10 minutes

1. In a large bowl combine the chicken, cucumber, and red onion and mix well. Add the cashew sauce and toss well to combine.

2. To assemble the wraps, place ⅓ cup of chicken salad into each lettuce leaf. Serve immediately.

3. The chicken salad can be kept in the refrigerator for up to 5 days in an airtight container, and added to the lettuce when you're ready to eat.

Per serving (2 wraps): Calories: 178; Fat: 6g; Carbohydrates: 8g; Fiber: 0g; Sugar: 3g; Protein: 23g; Sodium: 54mg

Time-Saving Tip: It doesn't take long to pull the meat off a rotisserie chicken, but you can substitute 4 (5-ounce) cans of chicken for the rotisserie chicken. Drain the chicken before adding it to the bowl.

Next-Level Elimination Tip: If you're eliminating nuts because they might be triggers, swap the Cashew Sauce for Balsamic Vinaigrette (page 182). It's a thinner consistency, so add only enough to moisten the salad—about ⅓ cup.

Baked Chicken Sausage with Apples and Potatoes

When buying sausage, it's important to make sure you choose a high-quality product. Look for sausage without MSG (monosodium glutamate) or BHT and BHA (preservatives), such as Aidells All Natural sausage. It is packed with flavor, with none of the preservatives you don't want. A good, natural chicken sausage makes this sheet pan recipe easy and guilt-free.

4 chicken sausage links*, halved

1 large apple, cored and diced

1 pound fingerling potatoes*, cubed

4 large carrots, cubed

1 large red onion, sliced

1 tablespoon honey

2 tablespoons avocado oil

1 teaspoon Himalayan or sea salt

½ teaspoon black pepper* (optional)

- **30 MINUTES OR LESS**

Serves 4

Prep time: 5 minutes

Cook time: 25 minutes

Time-Saving Tip: The size of the vegetables makes a difference in the cooking time. If you need the food to cook quicker, cut the sausage, apples, potatoes, and veggies into smaller, dice-size pieces and place them on two baking sheets. This will decrease the cooking time by about 10 minutes.

Substitution Tip: If you'd prefer, substitute butternut squash cubes for fingerling potatoes. You can buy them already diced in the refrigerated produce section of the grocery store.

1. Preheat the oven to 400°F. Line a baking sheet with parchment paper.

2. In a large bowl, combine the sausage, apple, potatoes, carrots, and onion. Drizzle honey and avocado oil over the mix, then add salt and pepper (if using). Toss well.

3. Arrange the mixture on the baking sheet in a single layer and bake for 25 minutes, or until golden brown. Serve warm.

4. Store in an airtight container in the refrigerator for up to 5 days. Reheat in a skillet or microwave on low.

Per serving (1 sausage link, 1 cup produce): Calories: 323; Fat: 13g; Carbohydrates: 42g; Fiber: 7g; Sugar: 17g; Protein: 11g; Sodium: 659mg

Tandoori Chicken Stew

This is easy and a crowd pleaser. Traditional tandoori is made with yogurt, but canned coconut milk makes a great substitute and cooks up into a creamy and filling sauce. The traditional Indian flavors are diverse and soothing to the palate. This recipe is a great one to double, giving you leftovers to freeze.

1 tablespoon avocado oil

1 teaspoon curry powder*

1 teaspoon ground turmeric

1 teaspoon garam masala*

1 teaspoon garlic powder

1 (14-ounce) can unsweetened, full-fat coconut milk

1 sweet potato, peeled and diced

1 large or 2 small broccoli crowns, cut into florets

4 chicken leg quarters, bone-in, skin removed

1 teaspoon Himalayan or sea salt

1. Heat the avocado oil in a Dutch oven or stockpot over medium heat. Add the curry powder, turmeric, garam masala, and garlic powder and stir until the spices become fragrant, about 3 minutes. Be careful not to burn them.

2. Add the coconut milk, sweet potato, broccoli, and chicken and bring to a boil over high heat. Cook for 25 minutes, then remove the chicken from the pot and allow to cool. Remove the chicken from the bone and add the meat back to the stew, then add the salt.

3. Gently rewarm the chicken on low for 5 minutes. Serve in a bowl as a stew.

4. Once cooled, the tandoori can be stored in an air-tight container in the refrigerator for up to 5 days or frozen in a zip-top bag for up to 6 months. When ready to eat, thaw in the refrigerator, then warm the contents in a saucepan on the stove.

Per serving (1½ cups): Calories: 415; Fat: 31g; Carbohydrates: 17g; Fiber: 4g; Sugar: 4g; Protein: 25g; Sodium: 773mg

- ONE POT
- FREEZER-FRIENDLY
- NEXT-LEVEL ELIMINATION–FRIENDLY

Serves 4

Prep time: 5 minutes, plus time to cool

Cook time: 35 minutes

Substitution Tip: If you don't want to bother pulling the chicken off the bones, you can substitute 6 boneless, skinless chicken thighs.

Caramelized Balsamic Chicken and Root Vegetables

The flavors of balsamic vinegar and honey create an acidic and sweet balance of caramelization on the chicken and veggies that will make you want to lick your plate clean. Chicken, a simple protein, is a good source of tyrosine, which is the backbone of all thyroid hormones.

For the marinade

⅓ cup balsamic vinegar

⅓ cup avocado oil

2 tablespoons honey

2 teaspoons Dijon mustard*

1 teaspoon garlic powder

1 teaspoon Himalayan
    or sea salt

For the chicken and veggies

4 boneless, skinless chicken breasts
    or thighs

1 large carrot, diced

1 turnip, diced

1 large beet, diced

1. To make the marinade, in a small bowl whisk together the balsamic vinegar, avocado oil, honey, mustard, garlic powder, and salt until well combined.

2. Place chicken, carrot, turnip, and beet in a zip-top bag and pour half of the marinade over them. Seal the bag and shake until well coated. Marinate for 30 minutes or up to 8 hours in the refrigerator.

3. Preheat the oven to 400°F and line a baking sheet with parchment paper.

4. Remove the chicken and veggies from the marinade. Lay the chicken flat on the baking sheet and arrange the vegetables around it in a single layer. Roast for 20 minutes, until all vegetables are easily pierced with a fork and the chicken is cooked through.

5. Remove from the oven and pour the remaining half of the marinade over the vegetables and chicken. Stir and place back in the oven under a low broil for 10 minutes, so the vegetables brown and caramelize. Remove from the oven and serve chicken and veggies warm.

6. Store in an airtight container in the refrigerator for up to 5 days. Reheat in a skillet or microwave oven on low heat.

Per serving (1 piece chicken, ¾ cup vegetables):
Calories: 358; Fat: 20g; Carbohydrates: 18g; Fiber: 2g; Sugar: 15g; Protein: 27g; Sodium: 628mg

Serves 4

Prep time: 15 minutes, plus 30 minutes or more to marinate

Cook time: 30 minutes

Cooking Tip: For best flavor, allow everything to marinate for several hours. The acidity of the vinegar penetrates the chicken and tenderizes it, while also providing an excellent flavor as it is absorbed into the chicken and veggies.

Substitution Tip: If you are not a fan of turnips and beets, substitute more carrots, or parsnips, red onion, sweet potato, or butternut squash. All pair well with this marinade.

Chicken Spinach Meatballs over Spaghetti Squash

This is not quite your typical spaghetti and meatball dish. But spaghetti squash is a nutrient-dense substitute for regular pasta. Avocado and spinach are good sources of vitamin E, which is beneficial to producing thyroid hormones. In addition to being nutritious, the green colors of the spinach and avocado are bright and appealing.

1 (4-pound) spaghetti squash
2 cups fresh spinach, firmly packed
1 yellow onion, roughly chopped

1½ teaspoons seasoning blend
1 pound ground chicken
½ cup Avocado Sauce (page 190)

1. Preheat the oven to 400°F.

2. Slice the squash in half, scrape out the seeds, and place it cut-side down on a baking sheet. Roast for 35 to 45 minutes. When you can pierce the outside with a fork, it is done.

3. While the squash is cooking, place the spinach, onion, and seasoning in a food processor and pulse until pureed.

4. Line a large baking sheet with parchment paper. Put the chicken and the spinach mixture in a large bowl. With wet hands so the chicken doesn't stick, mix the spinach and ground chicken until well blended. Form into 16 golf ball-size meatballs and place on the prepared baking sheet. Bake for 15 minutes, or until they start to brown.

5. When the squash is cooked, remove it from the oven and cool. When it's cool enough to handle, use the tines of a fork to "spaghetti" (scrape) the squash into a bowl. Toss each individual serving with the avocado sauce. Serve the meatballs over the spaghetti squash.

6. The recipe for the meatballs can be doubled and frozen after they are cooked. When freezing, place them on a flat plate or baking dish until frozen. Once frozen, place them in a zip-top bag for up to 6 months. To reheat, thaw in the refrigerator and reheat in the oven or microwave.

7. Store the cooked spaghetti squash and avocado sauce separately, as the sauce will begin to brown. Spaghetti squash will keep in an airtight container in the refrigerator for up to 5 days. Reheat in a saucepan. If you prefer, reheat it in the microwave in a bowl with 2 tablespoons of water, then add the avocado sauce and continue to warm.

Per serving (1½ cups spaghetti squash, 4 meatballs): Calories: 375; Fat: 18g; Carbohydrates: 36g; Fiber: 3g; Sugar: 1g; Protein: 24g; Sodium: 382mg

- FREEZER-FRIENDLY
- NEXT-LEVEL ELIMINATION–FRIENDLY

Serves 4

Prep time: 15 minutes

Cook time: 45 minutes

Cooking Tip: Bake the spaghetti squash in advance to save time. Once baked and cooled, it can be placed directly in the refrigerator for up to 5 days before using.

Substitution Tip: You can substitute ground turkey or pork for chicken and still have a delicious and healthy dish.

Turkey and Broccoli Skillet

The acidity of the lemon juice in this one-pot dish brightens the broccoli to the most beautiful color green, and adds a punch of vitamin C. Not only does the vitamin C help in developing hormones, but tyrosine found in turkey is the backbone of these hormones. This recipe is a great one to double, giving you leftovers to freeze.

1 teaspoon seasoning blend

1 pound turkey cutlets

1 tablespoon avocado oil

Juice of 1 lemon or 2 tablespoons lemon juice

1 cup chicken or vegetable broth

4 garlic cloves, minced

2 broccoli crowns, cut into florets

1. Sprinkle the seasoning blend evenly over both sides of the turkey.

2. In a large sauté pan or skillet, heat the avocado oil over medium heat. When the skillet is hot, add the seasoned turkey and brown for about 3 minutes on each side. Set aside.

3. In the skillet, combine the lemon juice, broth, and garlic and stir well. The lemon juice will help remove any brown bits left behind from the turkey.

4. Add the turkey back to the skillet, then add the broccoli. Stir and simmer for 5 to 7 minutes, or until the broccoli is bright green and begins to soften. Serve immediately.

5. Once cooled, the dish can be stored in an airtight container in the refrigerator for up to 5 days or frozen in a zip-top bag for up to 6 months. When ready to eat, thaw in the refrigerator, then warm the contents in a skillet on the stove.

Per serving (4-ounce cutlet, 1 cup broccoli):
Calories: 230; Fat: 5g; Carbohydrates: 14g; Fiber: 5g; Sugar: 4g; Protein: 35g; Sodium: 354mg

- ONE POT
- 30 MINUTES OR LESS
- FREEZER-FRIENDLY
- NEXT-LEVEL ELIMINATION–FRIENDLY

Serves 4

Prep time: 15 minutes

Cook time: 12 minutes

Time-Saving Tip: In the refrigerated section of the produce department you can buy bagged broccoli cut into florets. Frozen broccoli can be easier to use, but when cooked it will be softer than starting with fresh broccoli.

Substitution Tip: For variety, you can substitute chicken breasts for the turkey in this recipe.

Turkey Veggie Herb Burger Patties with Sweet Potatoes

These patties are a nutrient-dense version of a beef burger patty. They are packed with vitamin C from the bell pepper and iron from the greens and parsley, which help produce thyroid hormones. Aside from being nutrient-dense, the subtle flavor of parsley matches perfectly with ground turkey, giving this meal a unique flavor profile.

½ bunch scallions, roughly chopped

½ red bell pepper*, seeded and roughly chopped (optional)

½ medium carrot, roughly chopped

2 cups fresh greens, such as spinach, kale, or Swiss chard

¼ bunch fresh parsley

1½ pounds ground turkey

½ teaspoon Himalayan or sea salt

¼ teaspoon black pepper* (optional)

1 tablespoon avocado oil

6 baked sweet potatoes (see page 176)

1. Place the scallions, bell pepper (if using), carrot, greens, and parsley in a food processor and process until very fine but not quite a paste. You may have to use a spatula to push the veggies down to fully process them.

2. In a large bowl, combine the ground turkey, salt, and pepper (if using), then add the veggie mix and mix well with a large spoon. Use your hands to form the turkey mixture into 6 patties.

3. In a sauté pan or skillet, heat the avocado oil over medium heat. Cook the patties until they brown and cook through, about 3 to 5 minutes on each side. Serve immediately with a baked sweet potato on the side for each person.

4. Once cooled, the patties can be stored in an airtight container in the refrigerator for up to 5 days or frozen for up to 6 months. To freeze leftover cooked patties, place them on a baking sheet or flat plate and put them in the freezer until frozen. Once completely frozen, place them in a zip-top bag. When ready to eat, defrost overnight in the refrigerator. Reheat in a skillet on low heat until warmed through.

Per serving (5-ounce patty, 1 sweet potato):
Calories: 344; Fat: 18g; Carbohydrates: 28g; Fiber: 5g; Sugar: 6g; Protein: 20g; Sodium: 311mg

· FREEZER-FRIENDLY

Serves 6

Prep time: 15 minutes

Cook time: 10 minutes

Cooking Tip: When using a food processor, don't spend a lot of time chopping the vegetables. Chop them just enough to fit in the food processor and let it do the work.

Next-Level Elimination Tip: Bell peppers are considered a nightshade vegetable, which has the natural food chemical called solanine. This is a potential trigger, so if you're doing a next-level elimination of nightshades, just leave out the bell pepper from this recipe.

Eggroll Soup

If you love eggrolls, this soup is a deconstructed version—all the filling without the fried wrapper. It will hit the spot with its familiar and comforting flavors. The key ingredient, cabbage, is a good source of vitamin C, which you need to produce thyroid hormones.

1 tablespoon avocado oil

1 large onion, diced

1 pound ground pork

2 cups chicken, beef, or
   vegetable broth

½ head cabbage, chopped

2 large carrots, shredded

1 teaspoon garlic powder

1 teaspoon onion powder

1 teaspoon Himalayan or sea salt

1 teaspoon ground ginger

⅔ cup coconut aminos

2 tablespoons arrowroot powder

1. In a Dutch oven or stockpot, heat the avocado oil over medium heat. Add the onion and cook until soft and fragrant, about 5 minutes. Add the ground pork and cook until it's no longer pink, for 7 to 8 minutes, breaking up the pork with a wooden spoon so it doesn't stick together.

2. Add the broth, cabbage, carrots, garlic powder, onion powder, salt, ginger, and coconut aminos and stir. Increase the heat to high, bring to a boil, then reduce the heat to low and cover. Simmer about 15 to 20 minutes.

3. Remove ¼ cup of broth from the soup and place it in a small bowl. Whisk in the arrowroot powder to make a slurry. Slowly pour the slurry into the soup, stirring well, to slightly thicken the broth. Serve immediately.

4. Once cooled, this soup can be stored in an airtight container in the refrigerator for up to 5 days or frozen in a zip-top bag for up to 6 months. Reheat in a saucepan on the stove, until temperature reaches 165°F.

Per serving (2 cups): Calories: 401; Fat: 20g; Carbohydrates: 27g; Fiber: 4g; Sugar: 7g; Protein: 25g; Sodium: 823mg

- 30 MINUTES OR LESS
- FREEZER-FRIENDLY
- NEXT-LEVEL ELIMINATION–FRIENDLY

Serves 4

Prep time: 5 minutes

Cook time: 40 minutes

Time-Saving Tip: Instead of chopping cabbage and shredding carrots, buy cole-slaw mix, because the work is done for you. This makes this easy-to-prepare soup even quicker.

Cooking Tip: This recipe can be prepared in a slow cooker. Put everything in the cooker, stir well, and cook on low for 4 to 6 hours.

Sweet and Savory Stuffed Sweet Potatoes

This dish has just about everything. The apples and cranberries in the stuffing provide a hint of sweetness, but there's also a savory side from the sage. The apples and pecans offer a slightly crunchy texture, which contrasts with the natural creaminess of the sweet potatoes. Make this quick stuffing while the sweet potatoes are baking. When the sweet potatoes are done, slice them open, spoon in the stuffing, and enjoy.

½ apple, roughly chopped

½ onion, roughly chopped

¼ cup pecans*

⅓ cup dried cranberries

2 garlic cloves

½ pound ground pork

1 teaspoon Himalayan or sea salt

½ teaspoon black pepper* (optional)

½ teaspoon dried sage

2 eggs*

4 baked sweet potatoes
  (see page 176)

1. Preheat the oven to 425°F. Line a baking sheet with parchment paper.

2. In a food processor, combine the apple, onion, pecans, dried cranberries, and garlic and pulse until everything is very finely chopped but not pureed.

3. Heat a sauté pan or skillet over medium-high heat and add the ground pork. Cook for 4 to 5 minutes, breaking up the pork with a wooden spoon so it doesn't stick together. Add the salt, pepper (if using), and sage. Add the chopped onion and apple mixture and cook for about 5 minutes more, until the onions and apples begin to soften.

4. Remove from the heat and allow to cool for a few minutes before adding the eggs. Stir everything so all the ingredients are well mixed.

5. Cut a slit in the top of each baked sweet potato and squeeze the sides to create an opening. Spoon approximately ½ cup of the stuffing into each sweet potato. Put the potatoes on the lined baking sheet and roast in the oven until the stuffing is set, about 10 to 12 minutes. Serve warm.

6. Store in an airtight container in the refrigerator for up to 5 days. Reheat in the oven or toaster oven at 275°F.

Per serving (1 sweet potato, ½ cup stuffing):
Calories: 439; Fat: 23g; Carbohydrates: 36g;
Fiber: 6g; Sugar: 14g; Protein: 21g; Sodium: 611mg

Serves 4

Prep time: 15 minutes

Cook time: 25 minutes

Substitution Tip: Instead of using ground pork, substitute ground turkey or chicken, which may provide a leaner stuffing.

Next-Level Elimination Tip: While egg white is a pure protein, it can be a potential triggering ingredient. You can eliminate the eggs from the recipe, in which case you would not have to place the potato back into the oven. Without the eggs, the stuffing will be crumbly but still taste delicious.

Cinnamon Lamb Skillet

Lamb is a great source of zinc, and mushrooms are one of the few food sources that are high in vitamin D. Both nutrients are necessary to produce T4, the primary thyroid hormone. The addition of cinnamon, which is anti-inflammatory and high in antioxidants, gives the lamb a savory and sweet Middle Eastern flavor.

1 tablespoon avocado oil

1 onion, chopped

2 garlic cloves, minced

1 pound ground lamb

1 tablespoon dried oregano

1 teaspoon ground cinnamon

½ teaspoon Himalayan or sea salt

1 tablespoon balsamic vinegar

½ pound button mushrooms, cut in half

2 medium yellow squash, cut in ½-inch slices

¼ cup chicken or vegetable broth, or water

4 cups fresh spinach

1. In a large sauté pan or skillet, heat the avocado oil over medium heat. Add the onion and garlic and stir until they become soft and fragrant, for 3 to 5 minutes. Add the ground lamb, oregano, cinnamon, and salt and stir well.

2. Sauté the meat for 5 to 7 minutes, or until browned, then add the balsamic vinegar and stir well, getting the crispy goodness off the bottom of the skillet. Lower the heat to medium-low, then add the mushrooms, squash, and broth and simmer for 4 to 5 minutes.

3. Stir in the spinach and let it cook down until the liquid has cooked out, for 10 to 12 minutes. Serve immediately.

4. Once cooled, this dish can be stored in an airtight container in the refrigerator for up to 5 days or frozen in a zip-top bag for up to 6 months. When ready to eat, thaw in the refrigerator overnight, then warm the contents in a saucepan on the stove, until temperature reaches 165°F.

Per serving (2 cups): Calories: 375; Fat: 18g; Carbohydrates: 11g; Fiber: 4g; Sugar: 4g; Protein: 23g; Sodium: 338mg

- ONE POT
- 30 MINUTES OR LESS
- FREEZER-FRIENDLY
- NEXT-LEVEL ELIMINATION–FRIENDLY

Serves 4

Prep time: 5 minutes

Cook time: 25 minutes

Cooking Tip: If you prefer your spinach pieces smaller, use kitchen shears and cut the leaves into smaller pieces before putting them into the skillet.

Substitution Tip: Zucchini, sweet potato, or butternut squash make great substitutions for yellow squash in this recipe.

Lamb Shepherd's Pie

This twist on the traditional shepherd's pie is more nutrient-dense because of the addition of mashed cauliflower instead of mashed potatoes. By using lamb instead of the traditional ground beef, you are adding a good source of zinc that is necessary for making thyroid hormones.

½ head cauliflower, cut into florets

2 tablespoons avocado oil, divided

1 teaspoon seasoning blend, divided

1½ tablespoons arrowroot powder

1 cup vegetable, chicken, or beef broth

1 onion, chopped

2 carrots, chopped

1 cup peas*

1 pound ground lamb

1. Preheat the oven to 350°F.

2. In a large saucepan over high heat, bring 1 quart of water to a boil. Add the cauliflower florets and boil for 8 minutes, or until the cauliflower is tender. Drain and transfer to a food processor with 1 tablespoon of avocado oil and ½ teaspoon of seasoning blend. Process until smooth. Set aside.

3. While the cauliflower is boiling, whisk the arrowroot powder into the broth. This will be your gravy.

4. In a large sauté pan or skillet over medium heat, add the remaining 1 tablespoon of avocado oil, then sauté the onion, carrots, and peas until fragrant. Add the ground lamb and the remaining ½ teaspoon of seasoning blend. Stir to break up the meat and brown it, for 5 to 7 minutes.

5. Pour the gravy over the meat mixture and stir to combine. Transfer to a 4-quart casserole dish. Spoon the cauliflower mash over the meat and spread evenly with the back of the spoon.

6. Bake for 45 minutes, until the top is lightly browned. Serve immediately.

7. Store in an airtight container in the refrigerator for up to 5 days. Reheat in the oven at low heat or in the microwave.

Per serving (1½ cups): Calories: 485; Fat: 29g; Carbohydrates: 13g; Fiber: 4g; Sugar: 6g; Protein: 23g; Sodium: 290mg

· FREEZER-FRIENDLY

Serves 4

Prep time: 10 minutes

Cook time: 1 hour

Cooking Tip: This recipe can be divided into two 2-quart casserole dishes, so you can freeze one or both for later use. To do so, build the pies in two separate dishes using half the prepared ingredients in each, but don't bake them. Cover with parchment paper, then aluminum foil, and pop the whole thing in the freezer. When you're ready to cook, remove from the freezer and defrost on the counter for 1 hour. Preheat the oven to 350°F and put the casserole dish in the oven. Bake for 30 minutes with the parchment paper and foil, then remove and bake for 30 minutes more, until it's hot in the center and lightly browned on top.

Substitution Tip: For variety, you can substitute ground beef for ground lamb.

Beef Stir-Fry

Beef stir-fry is a simple yet sophisticated meal. Depending on what you're in the mood for, you can serve this dish with or without Cauliflower Rice (page 177). Beef is one of the foods that's highest in iron, and the vitamin C in bell peppers helps your body absorb that iron efficiently. These are both essential for thyroid hormone production.

1½ pounds bottom round steak or skirt steak, thinly sliced

⅓ cup Stir-Fry Sauce* (page 187)

1 tablespoon avocado oil

3 garlic cloves, minced

3 scallions, cut into 1-inch pieces

½ pound mushrooms, sliced

1 cup snow peas*

1 red bell pepper*, seeded and sliced

1. Place the sliced beef and stir-fry sauce in a medium bowl, and toss to coat the meat.

2. In a large sauté pan or skillet, heat the avocado oil over medium-high heat. Once hot, add the beef and sauce in an even layer and cook for 3 minutes on each side. Remove the beef and set aside. It does not have to be cooked completely, because you will put it back into the pan. Leave the sauce in the pan.

3. Decrease heat to medium and let the sauce simmer and reduce to thicken for 5 to 7 minutes. Add the garlic, scallions, and mushrooms and cook for 3 minutes. Add the snow peas and bell pepper to the skillet and cook for 3 to 4 minutes until tender.

4. Put the beef back in the skillet and stir to combine, evenly coating the beef and vegetables with sauce. Stir-fry a minute or 2, over medium heat, until the beef is hot. Serve immediately.

5. Store in an airtight container in the refrigerator for up to 5 days or in a zip-top bag in the freezer for up to 6 months. Reheat in a skillet or microwave oven on low heat.

Per serving (1½ cups): Calories: 353; Fat: 19g; Carbohydrates: 13g; Fiber: 2g; Sugar: 4g; Protein: 33g; Sodium: 259mg

· FREEZER-FRIENDLY

Serves 5

Prep time: 15 minutes

Cook time: 25 minutes

Substitution Tip: Feel free to swap out any of the vegetables and replace them with ones you prefer. Other veggies that work well with this stir-fry are broccoli cut into bite-size florets, carrot sticks, and water chestnuts.

Time-Saving Tip: To make this quicker, buy sliced mushrooms and minced garlic.

Creamy Beef Casserole

Casseroles are comfort food. This Creamy Beef Casserole is made with ginger that is soothing, cauliflower that provides vitamin C, and the gentle flavor blend of thyme and oregano. Double up the ingredients on the weekend and make a few casseroles that you can pop in the freezer to have ready-made dinners for the next several months.

1 pound ground beef

2 teaspoons seasoning blend

3 cups Cauliflower Rice (page 177)

1 tablespoon grated fresh ginger

1 tablespoon dried thyme

2 teaspoons dried oregano

2 cups chopped fresh spinach

2 cups chopped fresh kale

1 (14-ounce) can unsweetened, full-fat coconut milk

1. Preheat the oven to 350°F.

2. In a large sauté pan or skillet over medium heat on the stove, combine the ground beef and seasoning blend and cook until the meat is no longer pink and has browned a bit, for 5 to 7 minutes. Add the cauliflower rice, ginger, thyme, and oregano and stir to combine. Add the spinach and kale and stir until they're slightly wilted, for 3 to 5 minutes. Stir in the coconut milk.

3. Pour the mixture into a 9-by-11-inch casserole dish and evenly distribute the ingredients. Bake for 30 to 40 minutes, until the top is bubbling and browned.

4. Remove from the oven and let sit for 5 minutes before serving warm.

5. Once cooled, store any leftovers in an airtight container in the refrigerator for up to 5 days or in the freezer for up to 3 months. Reheat refrigerated leftovers in the oven or toaster oven at 275°F, or in the microwave. Frozen leftovers should thaw in the refrigerator overnight before heating, then bake at 350°F until warmed through.

Per serving (1½ cups): Calories: 268; Fat: 20g; Carbohydrates: 8g; Fiber: 2g; Sugar: 1g; Protein: 18g; Sodium: 98mg

- **FREEZER-FRIENDLY**
- **NEXT-LEVEL ELIMINATION–FRIENDLY**

Serves 6

Prep time: 5 minutes, plus 5 minutes to sit

Cook time: 1 hour

Substitution Tip: You can use any combination of greens, including Swiss chard, collard greens, or mustard greens. Any ground meat will also work, so feel free to trade the ground beef for ground turkey, chicken, lamb, or pork.

Cooking Tip: Get creative with the seasonings you use here. Aside from thyme and oregano, consider adding chopped or dried parsley, basil, marjoram, or rosemary to change or add to the flavors you enjoy.

Beef and Kale Red Curry

This "curry in a hurry" is an easy weeknight meal. Beef and kale are excellent sources of iron, which can give you a boost of energy if you are anemic, as often happens in people with Hashimoto's. It is also an important nutrient to produce thyroid hormones. Fish sauce is a common ingredient in Asian foods. It is a liquid made from fermented fish, important in enhancing the savory, umami flavors in the curry. Many supermarkets carry it, but if yours doesn't, try an Asian grocery store or order it online.

For the curry sauce

1 cup canned, unsweetened, full-fat coconut milk

3 tablespoons red curry paste*

1 teaspoon minced garlic

1 teaspoon ground ginger

For the beef and veggies

1 teaspoon avocado oil

1 pound ground beef

1 teaspoon minced garlic

½ teaspoon Himalayan or sea salt

½ teaspoon black pepper* (optional)

1 bunch kale, chopped

3 tablespoons coconut aminos

1 teaspoon fish sauce

1. To make the curry sauce, in a medium saucepan, heat the coconut milk, red curry paste, garlic, and ginger over medium-high heat. Whisk until all the clumps are gone, then simmer for 10 to 15 minutes.

2. While the curry sauce cooks, in a large sauté pan or skillet heat the avocado oil over medium heat. Add the ground beef, garlic, salt, and pepper (if using). Break the beef up with a wooden spoon so it does not clump. Cook for about 5 minutes. Add the kale, coconut aminos, and fish sauce. Cook for 5 to 7 minutes, or until the kale begins to wilt.

3. Pour the curry sauce over the beef and veggies and serve warm.

4. Once cooled, this curry can be stored in an airtight container in the refrigerator for up to 5 days or frozen in a zip-top bag for up to 6 months. Reheat in a saucepan on the stove or in the microwave.

Per serving (1½ cups): Calories: 433; Fat: 33g; Carbohydrates: 13g; Fiber: 1g; Sugar: 1g; Protein: 26g; Sodium: 670mg

- **30 MINUTES OR LESS**
- **FREEZER-FRIENDLY**

Serves 4

Prep time: 5 minutes

Cook time: 15 minutes

Substitution Tip: If you prefer, broccoli makes a great substitute for kale. Cut fresh broccoli into bite-size florets—or buy a bag of precut broccoli— and prepare it using the same method.

Cooking Tip: For the best-tasting kale, layer one leaf on top of the other (about 3 at a time) and cut out the spine using the tip of the knife. Then cut the leaves into bite-size pieces.

Unstuffed Cabbage Rolls

A quicker version of traditional stuffed cabbage rolls, this is an easy meal that can come together quickly. To round out your meal, serve this over Cauliflower Rice (page 177). The component in cabbage that makes it smelly—sulfur—is the same thing that makes it helpful for liver support. Since most of the T4 gets converted to T3 in the liver, it's important to support the liver through your diet.

1 pound ground beef

1 medium onion, diced

2 garlic cloves, minced

½ cup beef, chicken, or vegetable broth

2 cups tomato sauce*

1 medium green cabbage, cored and chopped

1 teaspoon Himalayan or sea salt

2 teaspoons dried parsley

1. In a Dutch oven or stockpot over medium heat, brown the ground beef, about 5 minutes. Add the onions and garlic and sauté for 5 minutes, until they become translucent and fragrant.

2. Add the broth, tomato sauce, cabbage, and salt. Stir well to combine, then cover and lower the heat to a simmer for 15 minutes.

3. Add the parsley and stir, then remove from the heat. Serve immediately.

4. Once cooled, this dish can be stored in an airtight container in the refrigerator for up to 5 days or frozen in a zip-top bag for up to 6 months. To reheat, heat in a saucepan on the stove or in the microwave.

Per serving (2 cups): Calories: 268; Fat: 9g; Carbohydrates: 23g; Fiber: 8g; Sugar: 14g; Protein: 28g; Sodium: 821mg

- ONE POT
- FREEZER-FRIENDLY

Serves 4

Prep time: 10 minutes

Cook time: 25 minutes

Time-Saving Tip: While traditional stuffed cabbage rolls have large pieces of cabbage, for this recipe the cabbage can be cut into whatever size pieces you enjoy. Larger cuts are more like the traditional recipe; smaller cuts are easier to eat. If you're going for smaller cuts of cabbage, you can buy precut coleslaw mix.

Cooking Tip: Sugar is a common ingredient in store-bought tomato sauce. When looking for tomato sauce, read the ingredients list carefully. You want at least the top five ingredients to be something other than sugar.

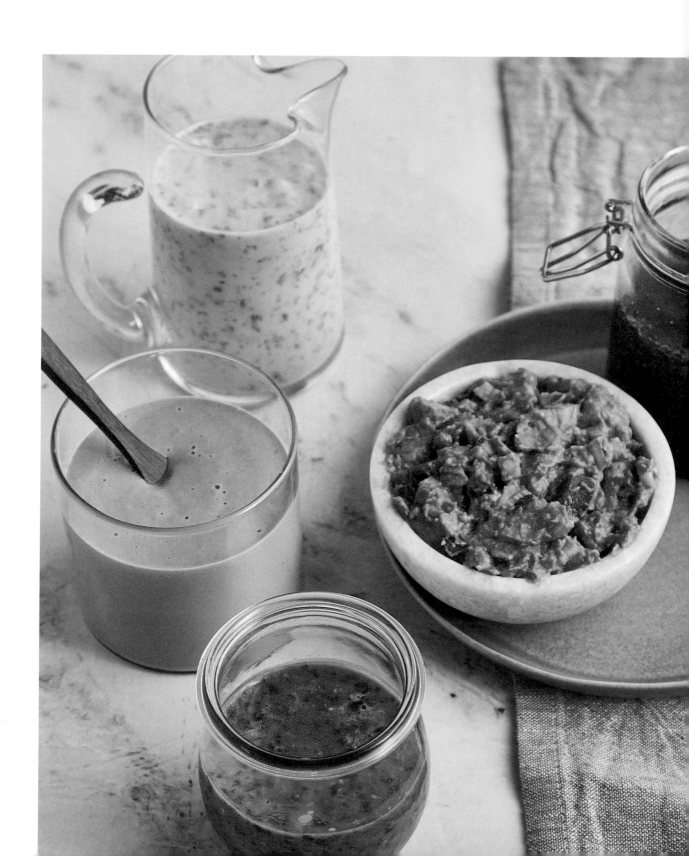

CHAPTER 10

Staples, Condiments, and Sauces

Baked Sweet Potato

Baked sweet potatoes can accompany just about any meal or be eaten as a snack. They are naturally sweet, yet they pair perfectly with savory dishes. Although they are complex carbohydrates, they are lower on the glycemic index and will not cause significant blood sugar disruption.

6 medium sweet potatoes

Pinch Himalayan or sea salt

Pinch black pepper* (optional)

6 tablespoons ghee

- ONE POT
- 5 INGREDIENTS OR LESS
- FREEZER-FRIENDLY
- NEXT-LEVEL ELIMINATION–FRIENDLY

Serves 6

Prep time: 2 minutes

Cook time: 45 minutes

1. Preheat the oven to 425°F and line a baking sheet with parchment paper.

2. With the tines of a fork, stab the sweet potatoes all over to help them cook more evenly.

3. Place the sweet potatoes on the baking sheet and bake for 45 minutes or until a fork can be inserted into the middle without resistance.

4. When ready to serve, split open the top of a sweet potato with a knife and season with salt, pepper (if using), and 1 tablespoon of ghee. Serve warm.

5. If you're saving the sweet potato for later, don't cut it open. Allow it to cool before storing. They can last in the refrigerator for up to 5 days. They can also be frozen whole in a zip-top bag for up to 6 months. To reheat, thaw in the refrigerator or on the counter and place in the oven at 425°F for about 10 minutes.

Cooking Tip: Always bake more sweet potatoes than you need and store them for easy use. This will make it more convenient for you to use cooked sweet potato all the time. Just pop them in the oven while you are getting dressed in the morning or when you are winding down in the evening.

Substitution Tip: You can buy sweet potato or butternut squash cubes precut and ready to cook in most grocery stores in the refrigerated produce section. Just decrease the cooking time to 15 to 20 minutes.

Per serving (1 potato): Calories: 232; Fat: 14g; Carbohydrates: 26g; Fiber: 4g; Sugar: 5g; Protein: 2g; Sodium: 111mg

Cauliflower Rice

Cauliflower rice has quickly become popular, and for good reason. Not only is cauliflower an excellent source of liver-loving nutrients, but it can be used in a saucy dish without having an impact on blood sugar. Both the liver support and stable blood sugar are a win when it comes to hormone health. This is a staple that you can always have in the refrigerator. Don't bother trying to grate the cauliflower yourself—just buy it already riced in bags. This recipe is a good one to double.

1 pound uncooked
    riced cauliflower

1. Heat a sauté pan or skillet over medium-high heat. Spread the cauliflower evenly in the pan without any oil or water. The idea is to cook out the natural water in cauliflower.

2. Allow it to cook and begin to brown on one side before stirring, about 5 minutes.

3. Cook until the cauliflower becomes browned throughout, about 15 minutes total.

4. Serve warm, usually with a sauce or stew over it.

5. Store in the refrigerator in an airtight container for up to 5 days.

Per serving (1 cup): Calories: 57; Fat: 0g; Carbohydrates: 12g; Fiber: 6g; Sugar: 5g; Protein: 5g; Sodium: 68mg

- ONE POT
- 5 INGREDIENTS OR LESS
- 30 MINUTES OR LESS
- NEXT-LEVEL ELIMINATION–FRIENDLY

Serves 2

Cook time: 15 minutes

Cooking Tip: For the sake of all things healthy, please do not steam your cauliflower in a plastic bag. When you do, the food will absorb some of the chemicals in the plastic bag. Cooking the cauliflower on the stove provides a better texture and eliminates the potential for toxic chemicals from plastic.

Time-Saving Tip: Using fresh riced cauliflower is quickest. However, if you have frozen riced cauliflower, allowing it to completely defrost will speed up the cooking process.

Plantain Tortillas

Bread and tortillas are often the biggest things missed when adopting a gluten-free diet. Enter the plantain. Plantains are starchy cousins of the banana. The green ones are less ripe, and therefore less sweet, which is perfect for these tortillas. These are a good staple for many meals, including the Ginger-Spiced Tuna Salad Wraps (page 129) or Nutty Chicken Lettuce Wraps (page 146).

1 pound green plantains (2 small)

⅓ cup avocado oil

⅓ cup water

1 teaspoon Himalayan or sea salt

1. Preheat the oven to 400°F and line two large baking sheets with parchment paper.

2. With a paring knife or the point of a knife, slice one end off the plantain, then run the point of the knife down the skin to cut it, and remove the skin. Cut the plantains into chunks.

3. Place the plantains, avocado oil, water, and salt in a high-powered blender and puree. You may need to start on a lower setting and gradually increase the speed as it blends. You may also need to scrape the sides down using a spatula during the process. Puree for up to 2 minutes until you create a thick, very smooth puree similar to the consistency of hummus.

4. Using a ⅓-cup measure, measure out batter into 12 equal tortillas between the 2 baking sheets, swirling them into circles with the back of a spoon if necessary. They should be approximately 6 inches across.

5. Bake for 10 minutes, then switch racks and bake for 10 minutes more or until the tortillas begin to form brown spots. Allow to cool before serving.

6. Store in an airtight container for up to 3 days in the refrigerator. They freeze well, too. Place a piece of parchment paper between each tortilla so they don't stick together, then carefully slide them into a gallon-size zip-top bag. They can be frozen for up to 3 months. Reheat in a toaster oven or skillet on low heat before serving.

Per serving (2 tortillas): Calories: 199; Fat: 12g; Carbohydrates: 24g; Fiber: 2g; Sugar: 11g; Protein: 1g; Sodium: 315mg

- 5 INGREDIENTS OR LESS
- 30 MINUTES OR LESS
- FREEZER-FRIENDLY
- NEXT-LEVEL ELIMINATION–FRIENDLY

Serves 6

Prep time: 10 minutes

Cook time: 20 minutes

Cooking Tip: The riper the plantain gets, the sweeter it will be. Adding a dash of vanilla and a sprinkle of cinnamon will enhance the sweetness. Riper plantains will need less water, so add it gradually as you may not need the full ⅓ cup.

Substitution Tip: In a pinch, substituting grape-seed or safflower oil for the avocado oil will work equally well.

Zesty Guacamole

Avocado is one of the few natural foods that are nearly pure fat. The fat in avocado is a good source of omega-3 fats, which is helpful to decrease inflammation. In addition, avocados are a good source of magnesium and B vitamins, which aid the body's natural liver detoxification process.

3 ripe avocados, halved and pitted

1 jalapeño pepper*, seeded and finely diced (optional)

½ medium red onion, finely diced

2 garlic cloves, minced

Juice of 1 lime or 1 tablespoon lime juice

½ teaspoon Himalayan or sea salt

¼ teaspoon ground cumin*

1 Roma tomato*, finely diced (optional)

- ONE POT
- 30 MINUTES OR LESS

Serves 8

Prep time: 10 minutes

Next-Level Elimination Tip: Jalapeño peppers, cumin, and tomatoes are all in the nightshade family and could potentially be triggering ingredients. If needed, eliminate these ingredients from the guacamole to make this recipe Next-Level Elimination–friendly.

Cooking Tip: A potato masher is a great tool to smash the avocados faster, while still getting the consistency you enjoy.

1. Scoop out the avocado flesh into a medium mixing bowl. Mash the avocados with a fork, making it as chunky or smooth as you desire.

2. Add the jalapeño (if using), onion, garlic, lime juice, salt, cumin, and tomato (if using), and stir together well. Serve immediately.

3. If storing, put the guacamole in an airtight storage container. Push it down with a spoon until there are no air pockets and it's flat on top. Add ½ inch of water on the top and store in the refrigerator for up to 5 days. When ready to use, drain the water off the top, stir, and enjoy.

Per serving (¼ cup): Calories: 114; Fat: 10g; Carbohydrates: 7g; Fiber: 5g; Sugar: 1g; Protein: 1g; Sodium: 123mg

Homemade Healthy Mayonnaise

Traditional mayonnaise is made with soybean oil. Even the ones that advertise that they are made with other oils often have some soybean oil in them. This homemade mayo is easy to make, but if you prefer to buy yours, review the ingredients list for *every* source of oil, and check for added sugar. Some of my favorite store-bought brands include Hain (made with safflower oil), and Primal Kitchen and Sir Kensington's (both made with avocado oil). Mayonnaise is made with raw eggs. If that's a problem for you, choose eggs that are pasteurized. Egg yolks are good sources of vitamins A and D, which are needed to produce thyroid hormones.

2 eggs*

1 teaspoon lemon juice

1 teaspoon apple cider vinegar

½ teaspoon Himalayan or sea salt

1 cup safflower oil

- ONE POT
- **5 INGREDIENTS OR LESS**
- **30 MINUTES OR LESS**

Makes about 1 cup

Prep time: 5 minutes

Cooking Tip: This can also be made in a food processor or a standing blender, using the food chute to slowly add oil.

Substitution Tip: Not all fats are created equal, so choosing fats that are less inflammatory is important. Other neutral-flavored oils you can safely use for your mayo include grape-seed oil, sunflower oil, light olive oil, or a combination of oils.

1. In a wide-mouth, 16-ounce canning jar, combine the eggs, lemon juice, apple cider vinegar, and salt. Using a handheld immersion blender, blend until well combined.

2. With the blender still on, gradually drizzle in the oil and blend well until it thickens. It is very important to slowly add the oil, because if it is added too quickly it will not emulsify with the egg mixture and will not thicken.

3. Store in an airtight container in the refrigerator for up to 7 days.

Per serving (1 tablespoon): Calories: 129; Fat: 14g; Carbohydrates: 0g; Fiber: 0g; Sugar: 0g; Protein: 1g; Sodium: 66mg

Balsamic Vinaigrette

Many salad dressings are made with soybean oil, which contributes to inflammation. This balsamic vinegar salad dressing is easy. It adds flavor to salads and can also be used as a marinade, as it is for Caramelized Balsamic Chicken and Root Vegetables (page 150). If you'd prefer a store-bought brand, review the ingredients list for *every* source of oil, and check for added sugar, soy, or gluten. Primal Kitchen or Tessemae's Balsamic Vinaigrette and Marinade are good choices.

2 tablespoons balsamic vinegar

1 garlic clove, minced

½ teaspoon Dijon mustard*

½ teaspoon Himalayan or sea salt

Pinch black pepper* (optional)

¼ cup extra-virgin olive oil

- ONE POT
- 5 INGREDIENTS OR LESS
- 30 MINUTES OR LESS

Makes about ¾ cup

Prep time: 5 minutes

Cooking Tip: You can also mix this using a blender or immersion blender for a quicker result.

Substitution Tip: For the oil base, you can swap avocado oil for the olive oil.

1. In a wide-mouth, 16-ounce canning jar, combine the balsamic vinegar, garlic, mustard, salt, and pepper (if using). Shake until the salt is dissolved.

2. Using a whisk, slowly add the olive oil in a thin stream until emulsified.

3. Store in an airtight container in the pantry for up to 2 weeks.

Per serving (2 tablespoons): Calories: 78; Fat: 8g; Carbohydrates: 1g; Fiber: 0g; Sugar: 1g; Protein: 0g; Sodium: 84mg

Citrus Ginger Cilantro Dressing

Lemon and ginger are the perfect duo, giving this salad dressing a refreshing zest of flavor. The olive oil in this recipe is a good source of monounsaturated fats that replace the typical soybean oil found in most dressings. This dressing pairs perfectly with salads like the Crunchy Tuna Salad (page 128). If you'd prefer a store-bought brand, review the ingredients list for *every* source of oil, and check for added sugar, soy, or gluten. Primal Kitchen Sesame Ginger Vinaigrette and Marinade is a good choice.

⅓ cup extra-virgin olive oil

Juice of 1 lemon or 2 tablespoons lemon juice

2 teaspoons honey

1 (2-inch) piece fresh ginger

2 garlic cloves

½ teaspoon Himalayan or sea salt

⅓ bunch fresh cilantro

- ONE POT
- 30 MINUTES OR LESS
- NEXT-LEVEL ELIMINATION

Makes about ¾ cup

Prep time: 5 minutes

1. In a blender, combine the olive oil, lemon juice, honey, ginger, garlic, and salt and puree until smooth.

2. Add the cilantro and blend on low until well combined.

3. Store in an airtight container for up to 10 days.

Per serving (2 tablespoons): Calories: 113; Fat: 11g; Carbohydrates: 4g; Fiber: 1g; Sugar: 2g; Protein: 1g; Sodium: 166mg

Substitution Tip: Substitute 1 teaspoon of ground ginger for the ginger root and 1 teaspoon of garlic powder for the garlic cloves for ease. If you're making this substitution, you may not even need a blender. You can whisk the ingredients together and chop the cilantro before adding it.

Cooking Tip: If you are not a fan of cilantro, this recipe is still delicious without it.

Ranch Dressing

Dill is the ingredient that gives ranch its classic flavor. This recipe can be used any way you would use traditional ranch dressing, including as a veggie dip, salad dressing, or as a dip for the Cauliflower Buffalo Bites (page 104). There is a variety of store-bought ranch dressings that are dairy-free and soy-free, including Tessemae's, Sir Kensington's, and Primal Kitchen.

1 cup canned, unsweetened, full-fat coconut milk, well mixed

¼ cup avocado oil

2 tablespoons apple cider vinegar

1 tablespoon dried chives

1 tablespoon dried parsley

1 teaspoon dried dill

1 teaspoon garlic powder

1 teaspoon Himalayan or sea salt

½ teaspoon onion powder

- ONE POT
- 30 MINUTES OR LESS
- NEXT-LEVEL ELIMINATION–FRIENDLY

Makes about ¾ cup

Prep time: 5 minutes

Cooking Tip: If you don't have a blender, you can whisk these ingredients together in a large bowl, or put everything in a canning jar and mix well.

Substitution Tip: Extra-virgin olive oil can be used instead of avocado oil and it will still taste like the ranch dressing you love.

1. In a high-powered blender, combine the coconut milk, avocado oil, and apple cider vinegar. Blend until fully emulsified.

2. Add the chives, parsley, dill, garlic powder, salt, and onion powder and pulse until well combined.

3. Store in an airtight container in the refrigerator for up to 1 week.

Per serving (2 tablespoons): Calories: 161; Fat: 17g; Carbohydrates: 2g; Fiber: 0g; Sugar: 0g; Protein: 1g; Sodium: 318mg

Spinach and Basil Pesto

This is a spin on traditional pesto sauce without Parmesan cheese. Replacing the pine nuts with walnuts adds omega-3 fatty acids, which are helpful for decreasing inflammation. This pesto can be used in a variety of ways, but my favorites include adding it to spaghetti squash or topping baked chicken with it to enhance the flavor.

4 cups fresh
   spinach leaves

4 cups fresh basil

¼ cup extra-virgin
   olive oil

½ cup walnuts*

Juice of 1 lemon,
   or 2 tablespoons
   lemon juice

½ teaspoon Himalayan
   or sea salt

3 garlic cloves

- ONE POT
- 30 MINUTES OR LESS

Makes about 1½ cups

Prep time: 7 minutes

1. Combine the spinach, basil, olive oil, walnuts, lemon juice, salt, and garlic in a food processor and pulse until the ingredients start to mix well. Use a spatula to scrape down the sides of the bowl as needed and continue to blend until smooth.

2. Store in an airtight container in the refrigerator for up to 1 month.

Per serving (¼ cup): Calories: 149; Fat: 15g; Carbohydrates: 3g; Fiber: 1g; Sugar: 1g; Protein: 3g; Sodium: 174mg

Substitution Tip: There are many different types of greens that will work in this recipe. Of course you can use only basil, but feel free to get creative and substitute kale, beet greens, or carrot greens to give it a slightly different flavor. I make a version of this pesto any time I have extra greens on hand.

Next-Level Elimination Tip: Walnuts can be a potentially problematic ingredient. They can be omitted from this recipe if necessary. It will still taste great.

Olive-Garlic Tapenade

Olives are a natural source of healthy fats that aid in decreasing inflammation. The anchovy paste enhances the flavor and is also a good source of iodine, which is the backbone of thyroid hormones. This tapenade can be added to salads, used atop baked chicken, spread on Sweet Potato "Toast" with Avocado (page 100) or spooned onto Zucchini Hummus (page 101).

1 cup pitted
 kalamata olives

3 garlic cloves

3 tablespoons
 fresh parsley
 or 1 tablespoon
 dried parsley

Juice of 1 lemon,
 or 2 tablespoons
 lemon juice

3 tablespoons
 extra-virgin olive oil

1 teaspoon anchovy
 paste (optional)

½ teaspoon Himalayan
 or sea salt

¼ teaspoon black
 pepper* (optional)

½ teaspoon crushed red
 pepper* (optional)

- ONE POT
- 30 MINUTES OR LESS

Makes about ¾ cup

Prep time: 7 minutes

Substitution Tip: You can substitute fresh basil leaves for the parsley to give this a slightly different flavor profile.

Cooking Tip: As an alternative to the food processor, you can use a potato masher to smash the olives and garlic into a near-paste consistency. If you're using this method, mince the garlic before smashing it.

1. Place the olives, garlic, parsley, lemon juice, olive oil, anchovy paste (if using), salt, black pepper (if using), and red pepper (if using) into the bowl of a food processor and pulse to combine.

2. Using a spatula, scrape down the sides of the bowl and continue processing until the mixture becomes a coarse paste but is not pureed.

3. Store in an airtight container in the refrigerator for up to 2 weeks.

Per serving (2 tablespoons): Calories: 90; Fat: 10g; Carbohydrates: 2g; Fiber: 1g; Sugar: 0g; Protein: 0g; Sodium: 354mg

Stir-Fry Sauce

Stir-fry sauce is traditionally made with soy sauce, which obviously contains soy but also gluten. Coconut aminos is an excellent replacement that eliminates both, and you won't be able to tell the difference. This sauce can be made quickly and keeps in the refrigerator for up to a month. It can also be used as a marinade or salad dressing. If you prefer store-bought sauces, some soy-free and gluten-free brands include Ocean's Halo Stir-Fry Soy-Free, and New Primal Classic Marinade & Cooking Sauce.

⅓ cup coconut aminos

1 tablespoon sesame oil*

Juice of ½ lime, or 1 tablespoon lime juice

2 garlic cloves, minced

2 teaspoons grated fresh ginger

½ teaspoon Himalayan or sea salt

- ONE POT
- 5 INGREDIENTS OR LESS
- 30 MINUTES OR LESS

Makes about ½ cup

Prep time: 5 minutes

1. In a small bowl or a wide-mouth canning jar, whisk together the coconut aminos, sesame oil, lime juice, garlic, ginger, and salt.

2. Store in an airtight container in the refrigerator for up to 1 month.

Per serving (2 tablespoons): Calories: 57; Fat: 4g; Carbohydrates: 6g; Fiber: 0g; Sugar: 0g; Protein: 0g; Sodium: 253mg

Cooking Tip: If you prefer a thicker sauce, in a small saucepan combine the coconut aminos, sesame oil, lime juice, garlic, ginger, and salt. Whisk together and heat over medium-low heat. In a separate small bowl, mix 1 teaspoon of arrowroot powder and 1 tablespoon of water to make a slurry. When the sauce is warm (not hot), slowly whisk in the arrowroot slurry. If poured in too quickly or if you use too much arrowroot, it will clump and have a stringy consistency.

Substitution Tip: Use 1 teaspoon of garlic powder and ¼ teaspoon of ground ginger if you don't have the fresh alternatives.

Cashew Sauce

The flavors in this cashew sauce meld perfectly, with the honey providing a hint of sweetness, followed by a kick of ginger. This sauce is great to use as a dip for vegetables, as a salad dressing, or in a wrap such as the Nutty Chicken Lettuce Wraps (page 146). Store raw cashews in the refrigerator until you're ready to use them.

¾ cup unsalted raw cashew pieces*

¼ cup rice vinegar

¼ cup water

⅓ cup coconut aminos

1 tablespoon honey

½ teaspoon ground ginger

½ teaspoon garlic powder

⅛ teaspoon cayenne pepper* (optional)

- ONE POT
- 30 MINUTES OR LESS

Makes about 1½ cups

Prep time: 5 minutes

Cooking Tip: The sauce will likely thicken after it's been refrigerated. Use water to change the consistency, adding 2 tablespoons at a time and stirring well to thin the sauce as you like it.

Substitution Tip: Instead of using cashew pieces, substituting peanuts or peanut butter will create a sauce that will be equally as delectable.

1. Put the cashews, vinegar, water, coconut aminos, honey, ginger, garlic powder, and cayenne (if using) in a high-powered blender or food processor and blend until smooth. Start with ¼ cup of water and add 2 tablespoons at a time as needed to make the mixture blend effectively and pour easily.

2. Store in an airtight container in the refrigerator for up to 1 month.

Per serving (¼ cup): Calories: 118; Fat: 7g; Carbohydrates: 10g; Fiber: 1g; Sugar: 3g; Protein: 3g; Sodium: 16mg

Teriyaki Sauce

This sauce is a bit sweet from the orange juice, honey, and blackstrap molasses, but it is nutritiously delicious. The orange juice provides vitamin C (make sure to choose juice without added sugar) and molasses is an excellent source of iron. Together they make a marinade that will increase thyroid hormone production. This is perfect for marinating chicken, fish, or shrimp and can be cooked down to make it saucy. For a vegan sauce, substitute coconut sugar for the honey. For a store-bought brand free of soy and gluten, look for Primal Kitchen No Soy Teriyaki Sauce.

½ cup coconut aminos

¼ cup 100 percent orange juice

2 tablespoons honey

1 teaspoon blackstrap molasses

2 teaspoons grated fresh ginger

3 garlic cloves, minced

- ONE POT
- 30 MINUTES OR LESS
- NEXT-LEVEL ELIMINATION–FRIENDLY

Makes about 1 cup

Prep time: 7 minutes

1. Place the coconut aminos, orange juice, honey, molasses, ginger, and garlic in a small canning jar and shake until well combined. Alternatively, you can use a whisk to blend them together in a large bowl.

2. Store in an airtight container in the refrigerator for up to 7 days.

Per serving (¼ cup): Calories: 80; Fat: 0g; Carbohydrates: 19g; Fiber: 0g; Sugar: 11g; Protein: 0g; Sodium: 37mg

Cooking Tip: If you prefer a thicker sauce, heat the finished mixture over medium-low heat. In a separate small bowl, mix 1 teaspoon of arrowroot powder and 1 tablespoon of water to make a slurry. When the sauce is warm (not hot), slowly whisk in the arrowroot slurry. If poured in too quickly or if you use too much arrowroot, it will clump and have a stringy consistency.

Avocado Sauce

Avocado and coconut milk pair perfectly in this recipe. This sauce can be used as a salad dressing, as a topping for fish or chicken, or tossed into spaghetti squash, such as in Chicken Spinach Meatballs over Spaghetti Squash (page 152). It is quick and easy to make and adds depth to anything it is added to.

1 ripe avocado

⅓ cup canned, unsweetened, full-fat coconut milk

¼ cup fresh cilantro

1 tablespoon lime juice

1 teaspoon garlic powder

1 teaspoon onion powder

1 teaspoon Himalayan or sea salt

- ONE POT
- 30 MINUTES OR LESS
- NEXT-LEVEL ELIMINATION–FRIENDLY

Makes about 1 cup

Prep time: 7 minutes

1. Slice the avocado in half, remove the pit, and scoop out the flesh into a food processor. Add the coconut milk, cilantro, lime juice, garlic powder, onion powder, and salt and puree until well blended. Serve immediately.

2. If storing, put the sauce in an airtight storage container. Push it down with a spoon until there are no air pockets and it's flat on top. Add ½ inch of water on the top and store in the refrigerator for up to 3 days. When ready to use, drain the water, stir, and enjoy.

Substitution Tip: You can substitute either avocado oil or extra-virgin olive oil for the coconut milk in this recipe. The alternative combinations will be less creamy but create an oil-based sauce that's great for adding to zucchini noodles or topping baked chicken.

Cooking Tip: If you are not a cilantro lover, simply omit it from this sauce and it will still be delectable.

Per serving (¼ cup): Calories: 117; Fat: 11g; Carbohydrates: 6g; Fiber: 3g; Sugar: 1g; Protein: 2g; Sodium: 475mg

Simple Hollandaise Sauce

Hollandaise sauce is a classic that can be used for more than just eggs Benedict. This recipe is great drizzled over grilled fish, steamed asparagus, or a fried egg. Using ghee in this recipe provides a good source of butyric acid, which is a healthy short-chain fatty acid used in the large intestines. We know that most of our immune system is housed in the gastrointestinal tract, so keeping our intestines healthy is necessary for keeping our immune system healthy.

2 tablespoons ghee, divided

1 egg yolk*

1½ teaspoons freshly squeezed lemon juice

Pinch Himalayan or sea salt

- **5 INGREDIENTS OR LESS**
- **30 MINUTES OR LESS**

Makes about ¼ cup

Prep time: 2 minutes

Cook time: 4 minutes

1. In a small saucepan, warm 1 tablespoon plus 1 teaspoon of ghee on low heat until melted, then remove from the heat.

2. In a separate small saucepan, combine the egg yolk, lemon juice, the remaining 2 teaspoons of ghee, and the salt. Place the saucepan with the egg yolks over low heat, stirring constantly for 1 or 2 minutes until the ghee is melted and the mixture thins.

3. Very slowly drizzle in the melted ghee from step 1, stirring constantly. Remove from the heat, continuing to stir for a couple minutes more. Serve immediately—this sauce does not keep well.

Substitution Tip: Instead of using ghee, you can substitute a good quality lard or refined coconut oil.

Cooking Tip: The egg yolk thickens the sauce and keeps the ghee and lemon emulsified. Use very low heat and stir constantly. If the egg yolk is overcooked the sauce will curdle.

Per serving (2 tablespoons): Calories: 142; Fat: 15g; Carbohydrates: 1g; Fiber: 0g; Sugar: 0g; Protein: 2g; Sodium: 124mg

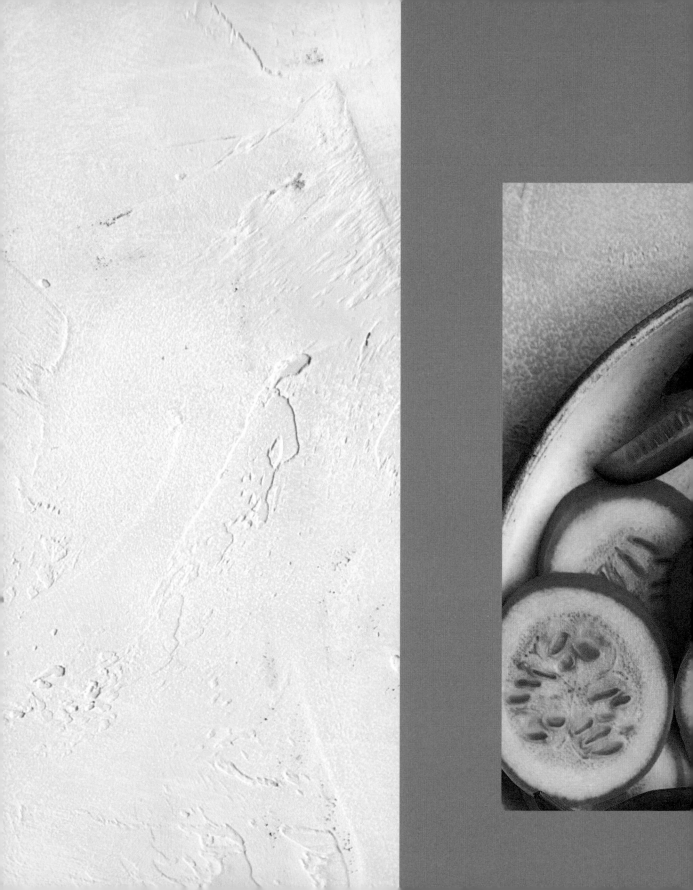

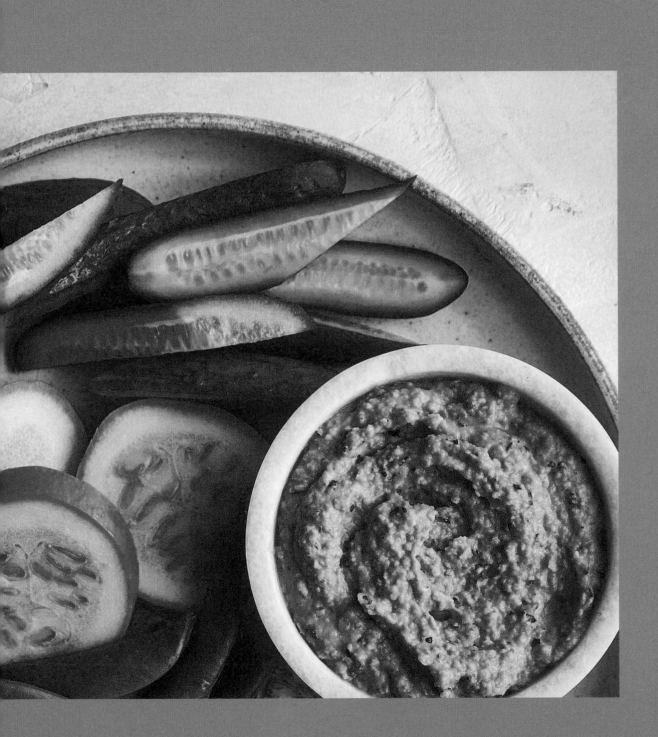

Measurement Conversions

	US STANDARD	US STANDARD (OUNCES)	METRIC (APPROXIMATE)
VOLUME EQUIVALENTS (LIQUID)	2 tablespoons	1 fl. oz.	30 mL
	¼ cup	2 fl. oz.	60 mL
	½ cup	4 fl. oz.	120 mL
	1 cup	8 fl. oz.	240 mL
	1½ cups	12 fl. oz.	355 mL
	2 cups or 1 pint	16 fl. oz.	475 mL
	4 cups or 1 quart	32 fl. oz.	1 L
	1 gallon	128 fl. oz.	4 L
VOLUME EQUIVALENTS (DRY)	⅛ teaspoon		0.5 mL
	¼ teaspoon		1 mL
	½ teaspoon		2 mL
	¾ teaspoon		4 mL
	1 teaspoon		5 mL
	1 tablespoon		15 mL
	¼ cup		59 mL
	⅓ cup		79 mL
	½ cup		118 mL
	⅔ cup		156 mL
	¾ cup		177 mL
	1 cup		235 mL
	2 cups or 1 pint		475 mL
	3 cups		700 mL
	4 cups or 1 quart		1 L
	½ gallon		2 L
	1 gallon		4 L
WEIGHT EQUIVALENTS	½ ounce		15 g
	1 ounce		30 g
	2 ounces		60 g
	4 ounces		115 g
	8 ounces		225 g
	12 ounces		340 g
	16 ounces or 1 pound		455 g

	FAHRENHEIT (F)	CELSIUS (C) (APPROXIMATE)
OVEN TEM-PERATURES	250°F	120°C
	300°F	150°C
	325°F	180°C
	375°F	190°C
	400°F	200°C
	425°F	220°C
	450°F	230°C

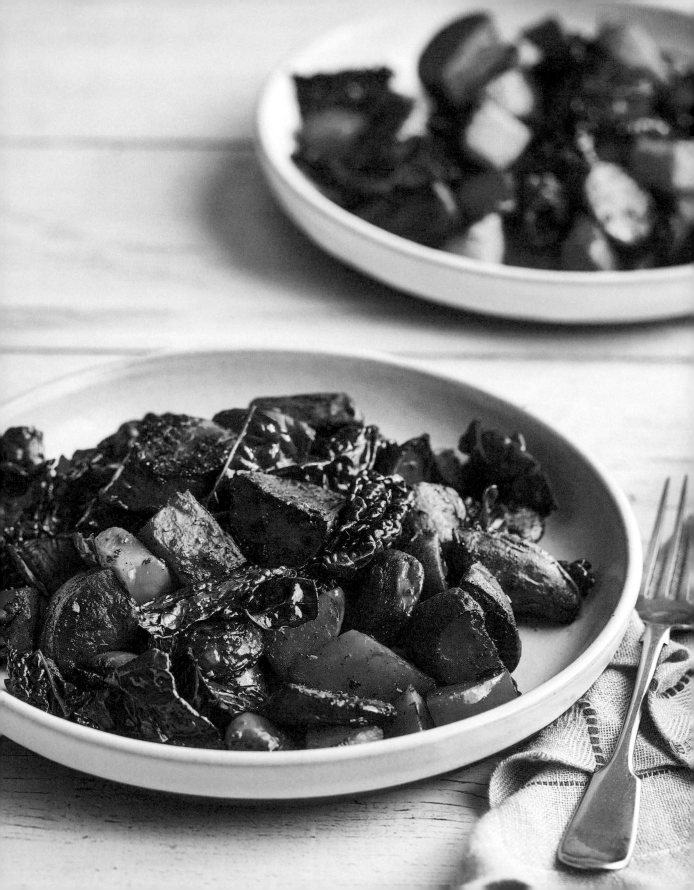

Resources

Recommended Brands

In this section, I've included some of my go-to Hashimoto's-friendly brands. These brands go the extra mile to include quality ingredients in their food, making them nutrient-dense without contributing to symptoms.

Canned Coconut Milk

Native Forest

> Found at Whole Foods Market or online at www.thrivemarket.com.

Natural Value

> www.naturalvalue.com
> Found at Whole Foods Market or online at www.luckyvitamin.com or www.vitacost.com.

A Taste of Thai

> www.atasteofthai.com
> Found at your local grocery stores and Whole Foods Market.

Thai Kitchen

> www.mccormick.com/thai-kitchen
> Found at your local grocery store.

Collagen Powder

Ancient Nutrition

> https://store.draxe.com/collections/collagen
> Found at Whole Foods Market, The Vitamin Shoppe, or online at www.vitacost.com.

Bulletproof Collagen Protein

> www.bulletproof.com
> Found at Whole Foods Market, Sam's Club, or Walmart.

Great Lakes

www.greatlakesgelatin.com

Found at Walmart, or online at www.thrivemarket.com or www.iherb.com.

Primal Kitchen

www.primalkitchen.com

Found at Whole Foods Market, Natural Grocers, Sprouts Farmers Market, or online at www.thrivemarket.com.

Vital Proteins

www.vitalproteins.com

Found at Target, Costco, or online at www.thrivemarket.com.

Eggs

Eggland's Best

www.egglandsbest.com

Found at your local grocery store.

Full Circle Market

www.fullcirclefoods.com

Found at Target, Whole Foods Market, or online at www.walmart.com.

Trader Joe's

www.traderjoes.com

Found exclusively at Trader Joe's.

Vital Farms

www.vitalfarms.com

Found at Target, Walmart, Whole Foods Market, or your local grocery store.

Avocado Oil

Chosen Foods

www.chosenfoods.com

Found at Whole Foods Market, Walmart, Target, or Costco.

Now Foods

www.nowfoods.com
Found at Sprouts Farmers Market or Natural Grocers.

Primal Kitchen

www.primalkitchen.com
Found at Whole Foods Market, Natural Grocers, Sprouts Farmers Market, or online at www.thrivemarket.com.

Coconut Oil

Barlean's

www.barleans.com
Found at Natural Grocers, Hy-Vee, and Whole Foods Market.

Carrington Farms

www.carringtonfarms.com
Found at Sprouts Farmers Market, Walmart, or Natural Grocers.

Dr. Bronner

www.shop.drbronner.com
Found at Whole Foods Market, Walmart, or online at www.vitacost.com.

Dr. Mercola

www.products.mercola.com
Found at Dr. Mercola site or www.amazon.com.

Field Day

www.fielddayproducts.com
Found at your local grocery store or online at www.luckyvitamin.com and www.vitacost.com.

Garden of Life

www.gardenoflife.com
Found at a grocery store near you.

Hain Pure Foods

www.hainpurefoods.com
Found at Whole Foods Market or Natural Grocers.

Kirkland

www.costco.com/kirkland-signature.html
Found exclusively at Costco.

Native Forest

Found at Whole Foods Market or online at www.thrivemarket.com

NOW Foods

www.nowfoods.com
Found at Sprouts Farmers Market or Natural Grocers.

Nutiva

www.nutiva.com
Found at your local grocer or online at www.thrivemarket.com or
www.iherb.com.

Ghee

Fourth & Heart

www.fourthandheart.com
Found at Natural Grocers, Whole Foods Market, and Target.

Pure Indian Foods

www.pureindianfoods.com
Found at your local grocery store or online at www.iherb.com.

Tin Star Foods

www.tinstarfoods.com
Found at Sprouts Natural Grocers, Whole Foods Market, and HEB.

Olive Oil

Bionaturae

www.bionaturae.com
Found at Natural Grocers, Whole Foods Market, or Hy Vee Food Stores.

Bragg

www.bragg.com

Found at Whole Foods Market, Natural Grocers, GNC, or your local grocery store.

Field Day
www.fielddayproducts.com
Found at your local grocery store or online at www.luckyvitamin.com and www.vitacost.com.

Full Circle Market
www.fullcirclefoods.com
Found at Target, Whole Foods Market, or online at www.walmart.com.

Jovial
www.jovialfoods.com
Found at Natural Grocers, Whole Foods Market, or Walmart.

Kirkland
www.costco.com/kirkland-signature.html
Found exclusively at Costco.

Napa Valley Naturals
www.stonewallkitchen.com
Found at Whole Foods Market or online at www.thrivemarket.com or www.vitacost.com.

Newman's Own
www.newmansown.com
Found at your local grocery store.

Spectrum
www.spectrumorganics.com
Found at Target, Walmart, Kroger, or your local grocery store.

Broth

Bare Bones
www.barebonesbroth.com
Found at HEB, Whole Foods Market, Costco, or online at www.thrivemarket.com or www.vitacost.com.

Bonafide Provisions

www.bonafideprovisions.com
Found at Natural Grocers, Whole Foods Market, or Safeway.

Epic

www.epicprovisions.com
Found at Whole Foods Market, Target, and The Vitamin Shoppe.

The Flavor Chef

www.bonebroth.com
Found exclusively on their website.

Kettle & Fire

www.kettleandfire.com
Found exclusively on their website.

Pacific Foods

www.pacificfoods.com
Found at your local grocery store.

Condiments

Primal Kitchen

www.primalkitchen.com
Found at Whole Foods Market, Natural Grocers, Sprouts Farmers Market, or online at www.thrivemarket.com.

Sir Kensington's

www.sirkensingtons.com
Found at Natural Grocers, Whole Foods Market, Target, or online at www.thrivemarket.com or www.vitacost.com.

Tessemae's

www.tessemaes.com
Found at Whole Foods Market.

Wholly Guacamole

www.eatwholly.com
Found at your local grocery store.

Yellowbird Foods

www.yellowbirdsauce.com

Found at Natural Grocers, Sprouts Farmers Market, Whole Foods Market, or online at www.thrivemarket.com.

Spices, Herbs & Seasonings

Frontier Co-op

www.frontiercoop.com

Found at your local grocer.

Herbamare

www.avogelusa.com/herbamare

Found at Vitamins Plus.

Simply Organic

www.simplyorganic.com

Found at Whole Foods Market, Natural Grocers, and Target.

Sweeteners

Lakanto Monk Fruit

www.lakanto.com

Found at Hy-Vee, Natural Grocers, and Fresh & Natural Foods.

Swerve Sweetener

www.swervesweet.com

Found at Whole Foods Market, Natural Grocers, and Walmart.

Apple Cider Vinegar

Bragg

www.bragg.com

Found at Whole Foods Market, Natural Grocers, GNC, or your local grocery store.

Napa Valley Naturals

> www.stonewallkitchen.com
> Found at Wegmans and Safeway.

Balsamic Vinegar

Napa Valley Naturals

> www.stonewallkitchen.com
> Found at Wegmans and Safeway.

Spectrum

> www.spectrumorganics.com
> Found at Target, Walmart, Kroger, or your local grocery store.

Whole Foods 365

> www.wholefoodsmarket.com
> Found exclusively at Whole Foods Market.

Understanding the Thyroid and Hashimoto's Disease

American Thyroid Association

www.thyroid.org

The American Thyroid Association is a nonprofit organization dedicated to educating providers and consumers about thyroid dysfunctions of all types. The information provided is traditional medical information to encourage you to have conversations with your doctor.

Dr. Alan Christianson

www.drchristianson.com

Dr. Alan Christianson is a naturopathic endocrinologist who writes extensively about the thyroid and the role it plays in the function of the whole body. He discusses in depth the role of genetics, and links thyroid function with adrenal health and blood sugar management.

Stop the Thyroid Madness

www.stopthethyroidmadness.com

This website offers an unconventional approach to managing thyroid diseases. It is a good resource for better understanding labs and medications, along with many other thyroid topics that are not often discussed.

Hashimoto's Thyroiditis: Lifestyle Interventions for Finding and Treating the Root Cause, by Izabella Wentz, PharmD

This excellent book outlines the multifactorial causes of Hashimoto's and unpacks the many ways to approach a treatment plan for yourself. Dr. Wentz has Hashimoto's and describes the step-by-step approach she used to treat herself. Her book is backed by excellent resources.

Cooking Techniques and Recipes

Autoimmune Wellness

www.autoimmunewellness.com

This is an excellent resource for recipes for the Next-Level Elimination Diet. These ladies have found ways to have the comfort foods we always want in a manner that will support people with autoimmune issues.

Kitchn

www.thekitchn.com

This website is an excellent resource for learning basic cooking skills. While not all recipes on the website are approved on this elimination diet, it teaches basic and advanced cooking techniques.

The Real Food Dietitians

www.TheRealFoodRDs.com

This website is managed by two dietitians who recognize the importance of real food. It has excellent real food recipes that you can begin to incorporate into your regular routine.

Index

Page locators in **bold** indicate a picture

Acknowledgments

Thank you to the people who have supported me along this journey. To my mentor, Sherry, who sees in me more than my internal boundaries. She pushes me to always live up to my potential. To my bestie, Jackie, who listens actively and acts as a sounding board for me. To my parents, Terry and Darla, and sister, Rebecca, who have always been my number one fans. Most importantly to my husband, Jonathan, who has always believed in me and supported me in even my wildest ideas. To my son, Alex, who inspires me to be my best every day. Thank you all for being such an important part of my life.

About the Author

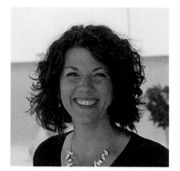

Daphne Olivier, LDN, RD, CDCES, IFNCP, is a food passionista, farm girl wannabe, and registered (yet unconventional) dietitian. She is also an integrative and functional nutrition certified practitioner, certified diabetes care and education specialist, and certified LEAP trainer, as well as the founder of her private practice, The Unconventional Dietitian.

From an early age, Daphne loved the idea of helping other people. As a young child, she knew she wanted to be a dietitian because she recognized the impact food can have on your confidence and self-worth. Later in life, she was diagnosed with Hashimoto's thyroiditis, so she understands what it's like to deal with imbalanced hormones.

In her practice, Daphne works with patients with varying degrees of metabolic and hormone dysfunction, including a wide spectrum of thyroid disorders. She is devoted to providing education, empowerment, and strategies needed to facilitate change, including nourishing the body and creating a healthy lifestyle. Daphne's goal is to help you enhance your physical well-being and gain confidence through the way you feed your body.